FEED
YOUR
SELF

What a compassionate and pastoral book! As Leslie Schilling dismantles the lies of diet culture in our world and in our churches, she also teaches us God's good plan for nourishment, embodiment, and even joy in our particular bodies. If you've experienced the damaging oppression of diet culture at the intersection of spirituality, this book is a healing must-read.

Sarah Bessey, author of *New York Times* bestsellers
A Rhythm of Prayer and *Jesus Feminist*

At a moment when entirely too many voices and images keep telling us what we should look like and aspire to, Leslie Schilling pierces through the noise and reminds us of what matters most. Oh, how I wish twenty-one-year-old Candice could have read this, but how grateful I am that *Feed Yourself* is in the world today!

Candice Marie Benbow, author of *Red Lip Theology*

One of the first steps toward living a life full of wellness is to confront shame and guilt with grace and the truth that we are liberated through God's unconditional love. Leslie Schilling reminds us that grace must accompany us on our journey toward healing our relationship with food and our bodies.

Dr. Terence Lester, founder of Love Beyond Walls
and author of *All God's Children* and *I See You*

Leslie Schilling has gifted us with a wise and beautiful book that teaches cutting-edge concepts about rejecting the lies of diet culture and replacing them with compassionate, scientifically sound alternatives that honor weight inclusivity, all of which is delivered through a loving and honest Christian lens. Every Christian who is interested in true health and well-being for themselves, their family members, and their communities should read this book.

Jennifer L. Gaudiani, MD, CEDS-S, FAED, founder and
medical director, Gaudiani Clinic, and author of *Sick Enough:*
A Guide to the Medical Complications of Eating Disorders

Feed Yourself is a deep dive into diet culture from a Christian perspective. It's not a book you forget about moments after reading it; it's a step-by-step, practical guide to gentle self-care that honors our bodies exactly as they are right now. If you know you want to move away from diet culture and need a faith-based place to start, this is it.

Megan McNamee, MPH, RDN, co-owner of Feeding Littles and coauthor of the *New York Times* bestseller *Feeding Littles and Beyond*

With warmth and honesty, Leslie Schilling guides the reader away from the "enemy" of diet culture and toward the understanding that their body has never deserved the shame and hatred imposed upon it. This book will be particularly meaningful for readers who have experienced food and body shame in the context of a faith-based community, which should have been a safe space in which all bodies can peacefully exist. By helping you reject harmful messaging and tune in to your inner voice, this book will help you reclaim a full, rich, and spiritual relationship with your body.

Paula Freedman, PsyD, licensed clinical psychologist, HumanKind Psychological Services

In *Feed Yourself*, Leslie Schilling writes from the heart with wisdom, kindness, and grace. The book's two parts allow the reader to fully comprehend the destructive impact of diet culture and then to create a path to healing and to the embracing of a peaceful relationship with food and body. Leslie's professional experience and connection to higher power and divine wisdom create a magical touch that is vital for unlocking the oppression of diet culture, freeing the reader to take the journey to peace and real health.

Wendy Oliver-Pyatt, MD, fellow at the Academy for Eating Disorders and founder of Galen Hope and Within Health

Leslie Schilling, RDN

FEED YOURSELF

STEP AWAY FROM THE LIES OF DIET CULTURE AND INTO YOUR DIVINE DESIGN

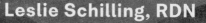

ZONDERVAN
BOOKS

ZONDERVAN BOOKS

Feed Yourself
Copyright © 2023 by Leslie Schilling

Requests for information should be addressed to:
Zondervan, *3900 Sparks Dr. SE, Grand Rapids, Michigan 49546*

Zondervan titles may be purchased in bulk for educational, business, fundraising, or sales promotional use. For information, please email SpecialMarkets@Zondervan.com.

ISBN 978-0-310-36655-3 (audio)

Library of Congress Cataloging-in-Publication Data

Names: Schilling, Leslie, author.
Title: Feed yourself : step away from the lies of diet culture and into your divine design / Leslie Schilling.
Description: Grand Rapids : Zondervan, 2023.
Identifiers: LCCN 2022060226 (print) | LCCN 2022060227 (ebook) | ISBN 9780310366522 (trade paperback) | ISBN 9780310366539 (ebook)
Subjects: LCSH: Reducing diets—Religious aspects—Christianity. | Body image. | Human body—Religious aspects—Christianity. | BISAC: SELF-HELP / Eating Disorders & Body Image | RELIGION / Christian Living / Inspirational
Classification: LCC BV4599.5.R43 S34 2023 (print) | LCC BV4599.5.R43 (ebook) | DDC 248.8/6—dc23/eng/20230422
LC record available at https://lccn.loc.gov/2022060226
LC ebook record available at https://lccn.loc.gov/2022060227

Published in association with the Gardner Literary Agency.

Cover design: James W. Hall IV
Cover illustrations: andipantz / studiogstock / iStock
Interior design: Denise Froehlich

Printed in the United States of America

23 24 25 26 27 LBC 5 4 3 2 1

To my family—
for riding the necessary waves
of unlearning and relearning

To C. C.—
may you live a fed and full life
free from the grasp of diet culture,
and may your generation do the same

Contents

Introduction 1

Part 1: Diet Culture Lies

1. It's Normal to Hate Your Body 17
2. Diet Culture Isn't in the "Safe" Places 25
3. It's Simple! Calories In, Calories Out 37
4. Health Equals Diet and Exercise. 47
5. It's Not a Diet—It's a Lifestyle 58
6. Your Weight Is the Most Important
    Indicator of Your Health. 67
7. Your BMI Is a Problem. 77
8. Health Lessons Teach Health 86
9. Your Weight Secures Your Righteousness 96
10. We're All Just Gluttons in the Temple 105

Part 2: The Surprising Truths

11. You Can Feed Yourself. 121
12. You Can Value Your Physical Health without Dieting . . .134
13. Pursuing Health Will Not Guarantee Health. 145
14. Mental Health Is Vital to Overall Health and Well-Being . 156
15. You Owe No One a Number on a Scale 166
16. Seeing Diet Culture Builds Resilience 176
17. You Will Not Look like the Influencer,
    Even If They Say So 186
18. You Can Detox from Social Media and Trackers 195
19. You Are You on Purpose. 205
20. You Can Choose Your Legacy 213

Acknowledgments. 226
Recommended Reading 229
Notes. 231

Introduction

I'm so glad you're holding this book in your hands. For more than twenty years, I've supported clients on their journeys toward food and body freedom. There are many lies that keep us from the truth. We are fearfully and wonderfully made, yet our culture has planted so many seeds of doubt in what should be the safest of places. But I am here with you. I'll stand in the garden right beside you, and we will pull every single weed of diet culture together.

What I Really Want You to Know Is—I'm Sorry

I close my eyes and imagine you sitting across from me in my office or in our Zoom rooms. My hand is on my heart, listening to your story. My response is likely different from what you expected. It may sound like this:

> I'm sorry you've struggled with trusting your body because someone withheld food from you as a child. For the confusion you must have felt when you knew you were still hungry but were told you had already eaten enough. Your body knew you needed more, but you learned not to listen to your body's cues.

I'm sorry you were forced to eat foods you truly disliked and couldn't leave the table until you finished. You may find it hard to even look at those foods today. This experience may have left you feeling sick and scared to trust your instincts. Your parents, caregivers, coaches, and teachers did their best. They just had no idea their comments would contribute to a lifelong struggle with food and your body.

I'm sorry you lost the freedom to be carefree in your own body because you heard your aunt speak hatefully about her own—the same woman you thought was so strong and beautiful. I am very sorry the pediatrician made it a problem when you grew bigger and faster than your sibling. I wish they had known the harm it would cause you.

I'm sorry you were told to "just be pretty" when you wanted to know and learn more. It breaks my heart that this led you to believe you are no more than a body to be decorated and observed. I'm sorry you were told to "stop crying and suck it up" when you were hurt and lonely—full of life and emotion. Love, you are not an empty shell—you are a whole person, body and soul.

I'm sorry you felt so much shame living in a growing and changing body. Your health providers forgot to acknowledge that your rapid weight gain was a natural part of puberty—your very wise body transitioning from child to adult. You deserved better.

I'm sorry you learned how to diet and engage in disordered eating in your middle school health class—you were just trying to do what you were taught. Far too often, these experiences lead to struggle after struggle with the scale and dieting. This is not your fault.

I'm sorry this culture—this diet culture in which we live—overvalues thin bodies and conflates body size with health, beauty, and worth. If you've carried a child, I'm sorry someone told you that you were supposed to snap back to your pre-baby body. This unrealistic pressure must have felt overwhelming after growing an entire human within you.

I'm sorry you learned in your church group that dieting and restricting your body from nourishment are righteous acts—*Jesus is the bread of life, but you'd best keep it off your plate.* It breaks my heart to know that a ministry leader supported such neglect of a divine soul. I'm sorry someone wrapped a diet plan in a Bible verse and told you it was God's will for you to live in a smaller body when bodies of all shapes and sizes are fearfully and wonderfully made. It makes sense how we got here—we all live in diet culture—but that doesn't erase the damage done.

I'm sorry a health professional said you had to count things—points, calories, macros, pounds—to be healthy. I'm sorry you received poor healthcare because of the color of your skin or the size of your body. I'm sorry you were led to believe your body is wrong and not to be trusted. Your body isn't wrong or untrustworthy. It was made to be so very wise.

I'm sorry seeds of doubt were planted in your soul so early in life, and that this was done without your consent. I am so very sorry.

But know this: together, we will do our best to uproot every single weed of doubt. And when that sly weed moves to the other side of your garden, we will pull it up again. We will root out every weed of shame and replace them

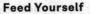

with seeds of truth. We will burn these lies to the ground and watch freedom rise from their ashes.

Body hatred and chronic dieting will not be our legacy. Beloved, this will end with us.

I Didn't Always Think This Way

I've been in the ever-changing field of health and nutrition for more than two decades, and let me tell you, I am beyond grateful that I've evolved. If you would have met me as a newly registered dietitian, I would have caused you harm.

I was a student of diet culture—all about the weight and calorie numbers, with no idea about the oppressive and powerful forces that influence real health and wellness. Learning about oppression, shame, trauma, weight bias, and self-compassion, to name a few, has grown me as a human being and a helping professional. I have a group of loving and seasoned therapists to thank for that. For years, they challenged, taught, and guided me to see beyond the plate. Today, it's less about the food and more about honoring the human experience and listening to the way diet culture has impacted nourishment and self-care.

I recently received a beautiful email from a client emerging from a life storm full of trauma and physical pain:

> I just wanted to say thank you for being part of helping me care for myself. It's been a year that I did not expect, and I'm not talking about COVID. The things I've been through made my heart feel like I wouldn't make it. Thanks for listening to non-food-related things at times and being patient with me. I don't think there are words or enough thank-yous to express how much I appreciate you. In the meantime, I hope this is

a new beginning for me, knowing I can allow myself to breathe, feel good about feeding myself, and regain trust in my body.

Had she met me twenty years ago, I don't think she would have felt the same way.

How amazing is it that we can continue to learn and grow in this world? We learn by the trials of life. We learn by the pain that others have caused us or that we've caused ourselves or others. And we learn by allowing interactions with others to help us grow. The unlearning and learning are continuous—there is no end to that exercise.

Although the idea of expanding our minds may sound exhilarating, it can often feel challenging and uncomfortable in practice. This tension is called cognitive dissonance, which *Psychology Today* defines as "the state of discomfort felt when two or more modes of thought contradict each other."[1]

From learning about diet culture in safe places—such as churches, schools, and medical offices—to understanding the true determinants of health to finding pleasure in eating to celebrating body diversity, it's likely this book will cause you to feel some cognitive dissonance. That's okay. Do your best to be patient and extend compassion to yourself as you explore these new ways of thinking and let go of long-held beliefs. Though this process can feel painful at times, maybe even agonizing, know that food and body peace are well worth the journey. You are not alone.

We All Live Here

A colleague was reviewing my last book and helping me make some revisions. I had written that most people are harmed by diet culture in some way by the time they reach adulthood. She struck that sentence and wrote, "No one gets out unscathed." The more I read her words, the more their truth rose to the surface. We all live here. And even when we don't see it, diet culture taints our day-to-day lives in many ways.

Living in a culture that confuses thinness with health and promotes restricting our bodies instead of feeding them takes a toll on all of us. If you were a fly on my office wall, the stories you'd hear from my clients might feel oddly familiar. As you make your way through this book, you'll read many client stories (please know that their names and some details have been changed to protect their privacy). I'm humbled that they've trusted me along my journey, and they have taught me so much. I want to introduce you to some of them now. You will hear more about their journeys throughout the book. And you just may find yourself in their stories.

MEET NICOLE

Nicole sent a message to my office saying that some friends at her church mentioned my name and thought maybe I could help her with her nutritional concerns. She really wanted to lose those stubborn pounds that had crept on through her early years of marriage and having kids. When Nicole sat down in my office for the first time, she said, "Am I going to gripe about these extra pounds for the rest of my life?" As my clients can attest, I said, "It depends."

Nicole had (luckily) never been told by a medical or health professional that her weight was an issue she needed to tackle. However, she had signed up for every single diet trend over the last decade, and she had the Facebook posts to prove it. She was sad. She was tired. She was obsessing over numbers. She was getting questions from her kids about why she didn't eat dinner with them. And she was running out of mental energy and money to spend on dieting. Diets had never worked in the long term for her, and she thought that maybe a dietitian could make her weight-loss dreams come true.

Nicole and I had a discussion about why weight loss was so important to her. When she got honest with me (and herself), her motivation had nothing to do with her health and everything to do with the way she thought she should look. Looking the part meant acceptance to her. She had heard her whole life that she'd have to watch her diet as she got older. Nicole was simply following the lead of others before her—friends, parents, church leaders. But this type of "follow the leader" ruined her relationship with her body, food, and family. She just didn't know she had another option.

Her next steps depended on what she decided. Would she stay true to the course of counting every calorie or trying every new diet? Or would she decide she was done with it all and finally feed herself? After digging into how she developed her beliefs around food, eating, and her body, she opted for the freedom of letting go of the lies of diet culture.

MEET RICKY

Ricky was a highly successful businessman. He told me he had worked his way to the top of a powerful organization and felt very accomplished in his life. But he just couldn't get control of his eating habits or weight. Now that he'd made it in his professional life, he wanted to feel like he was just as successful with his health. Ricky's doctor had made many comments about his weight and body mass index over the years and finally referred him to a dietitian. That dietitian was me.

When Ricky visited my office for the first time, he was surprised to hear me recommend that he eat more during the day, and not less. His work schedule took precedence over his eating. He'd work all day and crash when he got home. He was famished and felt like he could eat the kitchen table. He even jokingly told his wife he'd eat her too if she got too close.

Ricky had picked up health and wellness magazines over the years that told him eating less (and less) was the best plan for weight loss and health. That's exactly what he did. His pattern of undereating led him to chronic overuse of caffeine during the day, an overwhelming hunger in the evening, and poor sleep every night.

Like many clients, Ricky thought I'd have him counting numbers and stepping on the scale daily. I explained that, as a dietitian who practices a non-diet and weight-neutral approach, I wouldn't use the tools of a diet culture that had already failed him. Together, we'd focus on helping him have more energy to engage in behaviors that made him feel good, such as walking with his wife and doing some grilling after work. This approach removes weight loss and restriction as prerequisites for health.

Ricky and I worked together to help him plan for consistent nourishment, sleep, movement, and self-care. Because he had grown up in diet culture, he had no idea he could choose something other than a strict diet and exercise plan. He'd never known that health is made up of far more than just food and movement.

MEET TERI

When I first met Teri, she was very guarded. She eventually told me she had expected me to assume that she eats too much and give her the same "eat less, exercise more" advice she received from other health professionals. Teri had lived in a larger body her whole life, and her parents, classmates, and doctors never let her forget it. She had been taught that she had a weight problem, and that eventually she'd come to believe it herself.

When Teri gave me her medical and diet history, she said that whenever she'd go to the doctor, she'd get unsolicited diet and nutrition advice, even if she was just there for a bad cold. It baffled her that someone would give her advice with no knowledge of the way she eats or exercises. She had come to expect this kind of treatment and began avoiding medical appointments whenever possible. She ate less and less as well, but no one believed she had an eating disorder because of her body size. She had no idea that eating disorders can affect anyone with any body size.

Teri and I slowly started working on healing her relationship with food and her body. It started with knowing that her "here and now" body was good and that it deserved consistent and adequate nourishment. After a particularly harmful encounter in a medical office, she realized she also deserved a healthcare team that would not make assumptions about her health. Teri decided that learning about diet culture and how it had harmed her would be an essential step in her recovery.

All of these clients have something in common—the lies of diet culture had taken root at an early age. They all viewed food as the enemy, feeling they were either "good" or "bad" depending on their food choices. That made it very hard to disconnect their weight from their health and self-worth. But we surely were going to try.

As I've grown in my career, I've learned that it's essential to be clear about my nutrition therapy philosophy up front. Just the other day, I sent these words in an email to a prospective client:

> I like to make sure clients know my philosophy up front and that you're open to it. I'm a weight-neutral practitioner who uses a non-diet approach. That means instead of focusing on restrictions and weight loss, we focus on behaviors that can improve your relationship with your body, food, health, performance, and overall well-being.

The response is almost always similar to Nicole, Ricky, and Teri's: *I just didn't know there was a way to approach health or well-being other than weight loss.* Of course, it's okay to want weight loss or think about it. We've all been programmed to want it and believe it's the fix for all that ails us. It's a radical act in this culture to feed ourselves adequately when we've been taught to pursue restriction and control. But there's a different way, even in the midst of diet culture.

We all live here, and we can live better.

So Here's What You Can Expect

I've divided the book into two parts. Part 1 exposes the many lies of diet culture that have built a foundation of shame and body distrust we continue to experience. These lies have sunk into every safe place and into our core belief systems. In this part of the book, the goal is to peel back the layers of diet culture, exposing it all until nothing is left hidden. You will soon see it everywhere. And you won't be able to unsee it. It's hard. It's ugly. It may fill you with anger at times.

In part 2, we will rebuild after the insidious lies of diet

culture are out in the open, and we'll
do so by stepping into truth. The truth
about health. The truth about our
unique differences. The truth that diet
culture, with all its sneaky tools, doesn't
want you to know. The truth that a fed
life is the only way to make this journey.
These chapters will light the path to a life and
a legacy that rebuke diet culture, even when it
shows up in the safest of places.

> **A fed life is the only way to make this journey.**

    Many excellent books have been published about
diet culture and its means of influence, such as the
church, abuse of power, patriarchy, racism, marketing,
body objectification, and so forth. I will highlight these
books in chapter quotes throughout the text, as well as in the
recommended reading section at the end of the book, so if you'd
like to read more, you can. This book isn't a deep dive into every
historical aspect of diet culture; rather, it extends an invitation to
see the thief that lurks among us in the "safe" places, particularly
in the church.

A Word about Words and Professionals

You'll notice that I don't use certain words, or when I do, I
use them in nontraditional ways. For instance, I won't describe
behaviors or foods as "healthy" or "unhealthy," "good" or "bad."
This kind of framing dichotomizes how we think about behaviors and foods, which doesn't support us in making nourishing
or health-promoting choices.

    It's important to know that many people living in larger
bodies have reclaimed the word *fat* as a neutral descriptor.
When the term is reclaimed in this way, we attach no good

or bad value to it. It's like saying I live in a tall, thin, or short body. When we react to the word as if it's bad or an insult, we perpetuate the false thinking that fat bodies are wrong or bad.

In my professional circles, stigmatizing language like *overweight* and *obesity* is noted in quotations or written as *ov*rweight* and *ob*sity*. Bodies are meant to be very different—some big, some small, and some everywhere in between. When you see these words written this way, it's a deliberate attempt to note that I disagree with stigmatizing labels for human bodies but am stating the way they're used in our culture and in academic research.

Body diversity is divine and has always been a part of our world. We are all created on purpose, from our life's calling to our body size—God doesn't make mistakes. It may also be helpful to know that the terms *ov*rweight* and *ob*-sity*, which pathologize body size, weren't grounded in medical evidence. We'll dig further into that in part 1. I almost can't believe it myself.

Body diversity is divine and has always been a part of our world.

As you flip through the pages of this book, you'll see many stories not just from clients but from friends and family members as well. You'll also see stories about health practitioners, teachers, and coaches who have caused harm to others. Please know that I'm not condemning them. I've caused the same hurt and have been in their shoes. I'm condemning a system that sets us up to harm others.

Be aware that this book has unsettling and potentially triggering stories. These stories need to be brought to light to show the harm that diet culture can cause. Do keep this in mind as you flip through the pages, and take care of yourself.

Many wonderful practitioners exist out there, many of whom consider themselves non-diet or anti-diet health professionals. This is the way I now practice. This doesn't mean we're anti-dieter, anti-nutrition, or anti-health. It's quite the opposite. It means we care for humans in a way that doesn't focus on weight loss or restriction but instead offers health-promoting strategies that align with a patient's values. I hope this book will inspire you to find non-diet physicians, dietitians, therapists, nurses, trainers, and coaches committed to compassionate, non-stigmatizing, and "love your neighbor" kind of care. I pray you'll find someone to care for your whole self, not just about the food you put in your mouth or the exercise you do.

Throughout the book, I use the word *enemy*. It's important to share what that means to me. I didn't grow up using that language; it's just something that evolved in my mind over time. I believe there is evil in this world, which I consider to be *the enemy*. Diet culture is a tool of the enemy.

Different yet Together

One final note: I won't ask you to challenge your thinking on anything I haven't done myself. Over the last several years, I've had the opportunity to learn more about my unearned benefits in this life, as well as about deep-rooted systemic issues I hadn't known to address. I am now committed to lifelong learning (and unlearning).

That leads me to a necessary disclosure. I'm a human with many benefits. As a thin, straight, economically and educationally privileged white female, my lived experience may be similar to yours or very different from yours. I've never felt hunger from not having enough food. I've never experienced bullying or oppression because of my skin color or body size. Though I may not know what it's like to live in your body or to experience your life, I've been fortunate to learn about and be challenged by the experiences that clients, colleagues, and friends have shared with me.

We all navigate the world with differing circumstances, but we share life in this Western culture, which is a diet- and body-obsessed society. Even though I'm a dietitian with specialties in eating disorders and sports nutrition, I grew up swimming in the waters of diet culture. I am not immune to the lies that keep us stuck in body dissatisfaction and oppression. We all have tough days; it's part of being human. But hopefully, once our eyes are opened to these diet culture lies, we can begin fighting and building resilience against them.

As you work through each part of this book, please know that I'm praying you will read each chapter with curiosity and compassion for yourself, your neighbor, and your journey. I want you to know that I'm genuinely sorry for the lies you were told about your body and the bodies of others. Let's break these chains together.

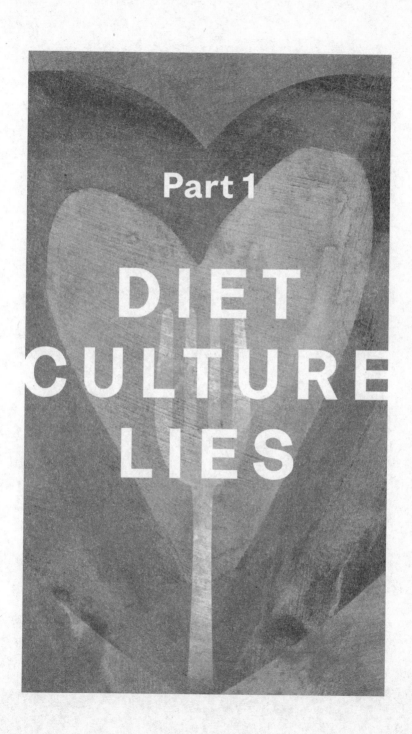

Part 1

DIET CULTURE LIES

It's Normal to Hate Your Body

> Oh my God, what if you wake up some day, and you're 65 or 75, and you never got your memoir or novel written; or you didn't go swimming in warm pools and oceans all those years because your thighs were jiggly and you had a nice big comfortable tummy; or you were just so strung out on perfectionism and people-pleasing that you forgot to have a big juicy creative life, of imagination and radical silliness and staring off into space like when you were a kid? It's going to break your heart. Don't let this happen.
>
> **Anne Lamott, Facebook post, May 12, 2014**

Kate wouldn't speak. She just let the tears run down her face as she sat in my counseling office. Her mom quickly took over the session, saying with great disappointment something to the effect, "Just look at her." Her mom—we'll call her Linda—was put together from head to toe. Linda wore a spectacular outfit, her makeup shimmered, her nails were perfectly manicured, and not a hair was out of place. Her daughter was a stark contrast. Linda was interested in one thing—changing Kate's body before she left for college.

Linda went on to say that there was no way anyone would ever find her daughter attractive with chipped nails, a bad diet, and a body like the one she had. Tears filled my eyes. My heart broke for her. It hurts for everyone who hears the message that they're not enough from a loved one, from our culture, and then, of course, from themselves.

This is one of the many reasons I have tissues in my office. When we talk about food and our bodies, we open a door to deep vulnerability. Sometimes that door leads us to body confidence and autonomy, but in my professional experience, it most often leads to hallways of shame and doubt. We long to feel unbroken and good enough. Our culture teaches the false truth that changing our bodies is the fix. Although food is often perceived as the culprit, it's rarely the problem; rather, the problem is we're taught that hating our bodies is part of the human experience. Body hatred is learned—it is not innate.

Do You Remember the Moment?

Do you remember the moment when you first questioned whether or not your body was good? The moment you wondered if eating this or that food was good or bad? Think back to your childhood or early teen years. Think back to the early influences in your life—parents, grandparents, teachers, Sunday school leaders, Uncle Bob, siblings, friends, maybe even a pastor or pediatrician. Think about all of the people in your circle of trust. People you loved. People who loved you. People who, deep down, only wanted what was best for you. Not all of our moments look as stark and overt as Kate's looked. Some are much subtler, building significant distress and doubt over months and years until we're swimming in self-doubt. Either way, most of us living in this body-obsessed culture have a moment like this.

Are you sure you want to eat that? Won't that mess up your diet? Is that really the size you want? Aren't you trying to lose weight? It would be best if you didn't eat that snack. Maybe you should try Weight Watchers. These were the words of caution my mother, sister, and I regularly heard from my grandmother growing up. Many adored and looked up to my God-fearing, strong-willed, wartime turned polio-epidemic nurse of a grandmother. What an amazing woman she was! Oh, how I loved Mabel.

Nanny (that's what we called her) would always write the menu for our visit on a white paper plate by the stove in her kitchen. As soon as we'd get to her house, I'd run into the kitchen and climb up on the black vinyl–cushioned stool in the corner to see what delicious plans Nanny had penciled in for our meal. My entrepreneurial spirit and love of planning meals most likely came from her. My early distrust of the body I was living in also came from her. I had no idea body hatred was a legacy I didn't have to accept, and you don't have to accept it either.

None of This Was Nanny's Fault

None of this was Nanny's fault, and it wasn't Kate's mom's fault either. For generations, humans (not a loving God) attempting to earn God's grace set a bar of earthly purity so high that we were doomed to fail. It makes sense that we're here—at the crossroad between a legacy that was and a legacy that no longer has to be. The struggle dates back to the Garden of Eden and Adam and Eve's first family. After the fall, Adam and Eve covered their nakedness and felt shame for the first time (see Genesis 3). They had concerns about their bodies and food that they'd never had before.

The early Christian church was profoundly influenced by Roman culture. Rome (around the time of the apostle Paul's letters) was a culture driven by patriarchy. In those times, if you weren't a man, you were the property of one. We still see various shades of this in our culture.

The idea of the objectification of women didn't end in the first century. Some churches even today suggest that keeping a trim body and maintaining attractiveness for the husband's benefit is a godly activity, maybe even a calling. Need a little help being obedient? Never fear; diet schemes wrapped in a Bible verse with a side of extra prayer can help you get there. It's no wonder Kate's mom and Nanny felt the way they did—the church family in which they'd spent their whole life preached it.

It's Not Only an Anti-Grace Message; It's a Dangerous One

Years ago, a newly married couple walked into my office. Having just been diagnosed with a life-threatening eating disorder, the young woman sat silently. She had very little energy, not even enough to speak. On the other hand, her husband was concerned that she might not be able to continue the highly restrictive diet their congregation was doing together. He didn't yet understand that this churchwide diet could kill her. It wasn't my first experience with a patient suffering from an eating disorder, but it was my first experience of a church that practiced and promoted one.

Dieting, which is a common and seemingly benign practice, is *disordered eating*. Our diet-crazed and body-obsessed culture has become intertwined with the church—it's a dangerous pairing of the secular and the sacred. How can we hate a body divinely designed for our unique walk in life? We aren't born with body hatred; as I said earlier, we learn it, even in "safe" places such as the church.

> Dieting, which is a common and seemingly benign practice, is **disordered eating.**

It's not a new thing for places of worship to promote particular ways of eating. You can find food rules, body shaming, and diet plans wrapped in an out-of-context Bible verse in almost every congregation in America. I get it. I used to think of dietary purity as my Christian duty as well. It seemed like a legitimate way to depend on God more and even grow stronger in my faith. I even believed it until I saw how this approach was wrecking believers—their lives, health, relationships, and families. I saw believers look down on one another because of the food they ate or didn't eat. I watched as church members praised my friend for her weight loss as she was dying from cancer.

After years of witnessing this hurt and harm, I experienced another very different moment—the moment I realized, as both a lifelong Christian and a longtime nutrition professional, that dieting to gain worth and offering pretend grace for one another were nothing but lies.

Christian values such as "love your neighbor," "don't judge one another," "don't covet," and "care for the least of these" have collided with a culture profoundly strung out on appearances, healthism, and perfectionism. Given this culture's false definition of health, the value of thinness falls seamlessly into the purity culture of many churches. After all, this is what the medical field deems healthy, right? You have pink eye—lose weight. Oh, you need a flu shot—lose weight too. Just here for some lab work—let's see what you weigh, which is a 180-degree shaming diversion from the real health issue that needs attention.

The "thin ideal," or the thought that everyone can just work hard enough and be thin, is the Western world's ideal. Not only is it untrue (much more on that later); it's also incongruent with our divine design. When we deny our bodies, aren't we also denying that we are made in the image of God—the God who knows each one of us? I believe that just as we have different colors of skin, speak various languages, and have vastly diverse shoe sizes, we are also meant to live in bodies of all shapes, sizes, and abilities. Not one human of any color, tongue, size, or range of ability is a mistake.

> We are meant to live in bodies of **all shapes,** sizes, and abilities. Not one human of any color, tongue, size, or range of ability is a mistake.

The belief that it's normal to hate your body is manufactured—a lie handed down from generation to generation. It becomes a cyclical trauma. The experience of being at war with our bodies doesn't have to be passed down like a family heirloom. There's a truth you can claim instead—namely, that your body was made just for you by the God of love, no matter what the world says.

I lost touch with Kate eventually, but I'm confident she knew her worth by the time she left home, and it had nothing to do with her body. Kate learned this truth over the year we worked together. She realized that some of her family's beliefs around food, body, and appearance were not her own beliefs. The year before she left home was filled with challenges, such as letting her family know she didn't want them to comment on her body (or food or clothes or fingernails); instead, she wanted them to support her to produce the best college application essays she could create. She also decided that instead of accepting the heirloom of constant body scrutiny, she would nourish her body in a way that supported her view of health, her dreams, and her divine uniqueness.

As I got older, I learned that Nanny did the best she could with the information she had. I was fortunate that I didn't retain the food or body shame she had carried her entire life. My path led me here—to wrestling with our culture, my weight-centric professional training, and an inescapable calling to speak truth to these lies. I tried to put this message to rest and just move on with my life many times, but God wouldn't have it. So here we are, friends, on this journey together. Let's expose the lies of diet culture. I promise you'll find paths to truth, grace, and healing on the other side.

THE WORLD SAYS . . .

If you change your body, you will be happy and loved.

THE WORD SAYS . . .

Do not conform to the pattern of this world, but be transformed by the renewing of your mind. Then you will be able to test and approve what God's will is—God's good, pleasing and perfect will.

Romans 12:2

STEPPING AWAY FROM LIES

Take a few moments to think about the messages you heard about bodies growing up.

- Were they favorable toward all types of bodies? Did they shame those in larger bodies?

- Was weight loss or thinness praised? If so, how did this make you feel?

- Did you have a moment or turning point when your environment or our culture made you question whether your body was good?

- Do you remember comments about bodies in your home? Your school? Your church or from believers?

- As you reflect on Romans 12:2, what do you think of the ideas you've absorbed about bodies through the years?

- Are you willing to investigate how many of these beliefs could be lies? Let's begin to replace them with truth.

Diet Culture Isn't in the "Safe" Places

> Culture can be wonderfully enriching. It can also be full of arrogance, prejudice, and division, so we must pay close attention and use our power and abilities to see and to think before swallowing the messages of our culture whole.
>
> **Diane Langberg, *Redeeming Power***

My husband gave me a pleading stare—like, please don't raise your hand, scream, or walk out in the middle of this sermon. He knows me. He knows what happens in my brain and heart when I hear body shaming—particularly from the pulpit.

I grew up in the church—the kind of church where saying you didn't have anything to wear that looked nice enough might get you a pass to skip a Sunday service. I learned a lot about God, Jesus, and the Holy Spirit in that little church. It laid the foundation for my relationship with Jesus today, and

I'm grateful. But back then, I also sensed that a person needed to look a certain way to attend church. Of course, I know that had to do with our culture and not God. But that feeling stuck with me for a long time—everyone must look the part to be a Christian.

I've since learned that God cares far more about the state of our hearts than about how much we weigh or what we wear. But I'm often reminded that the church is made of people living in a culture that elevates the value of appearance. And even pastors and ministry leaders feel the pressure. After all, they're as human and imperfect as the rest of us.

As I've developed in my faith, I've listened to many pastors deliver powerful messages based on the Gospels rather than on what our culture teaches us. On the other hand, I've also witnessed church leaders bring loads of food to the stage and talk about how awful they were for desiring it, or joke about wishing they had the same illness as that friend who lost a lot of weight. When a pastor suggests such things, my heart aches. I hurt for the pastor who believes those words. I hurt for the believers who question their choices around food and their bodies.

Food- and body-shaming messages from the pulpit aren't new. Our culture suggests that it's normal to feel dread and distrust around our bodies. It seems like an illustration from the pulpit that almost everyone will understand—a communal commiseration over our earthly vessels. Nearly every pastor or ministry influencer I've witnessed has used this approach in some way. The congregation simultaneously laughs and hurts.

The pastors I've seen preach have often been eloquent and humorous. On the day that my husband gave me the "don't run" glare, one of my favorite leaders was preaching. I braced myself as he started sharing thoughts about his own body and what that might mean as a Christian. As he delivered this beautiful, thoughtful, and funny message, he threw in this statement: "Maybe I won't be ov*rweight in heaven." My heart broke into a million pieces—sadly, the same way it had many times before.

All humans made in God's image are fully loved by God, no matter what a scale or clothing size may read. How fortunate are we to have the chance to fully receive the truth that we are fearfully and wonderfully made? Sadly, that truth doesn't keep shaming comments from sneaking into the church. We hope the church will be different—full of gospel grace and kindness and void of this world's commitment to diet culture. But we have an idol issue so crafty that it's practically invisible, even to ministry leaders.

A statement like the one I heard projected from a church stage led me to believe that this pastor may feel that his own body isn't good enough—just as many people in his congregation feel. Was he disappointed in the body that was divinely provided to him? And if he felt this way and made comments about the shame he felt regarding his body, what might be happening in the minds and hearts of those in the congregation? I know in my heart of hearts that this pastor meant no harm. Still, I believe that almost every person in that congregation reinforced a common untruth that day: if I live in a larger body or end up in a larger body, I am unworthy and I must do something about it. But I don't believe this is true. Won't all the amazingly different bodies created by God be in heaven? Every type of body will be celebrated. While there will be no more pain, there will be body diversity and proof of life. How are Jesus' resurrected scars not evidence of this?

O diet culture, you thief of joy, how you have tricked us. We must bring to light any and every piece of diet culture lurking in our safe places, but we *must* obliterate diet culture in our places of worship. This war we wage against our bodies is

The enemy can't win our souls, but he can most definitely distract us from our purpose by keeping us focused on shrinking our bodies.

so intertwined with what we wrongly perceive to represent righteousness and health that we don't see its toll on our lives, families, purpose, and potential. We don't see diet culture as spiritual warfare, but that's precisely what it is. The enemy can't win our souls, but he can most definitely distract us from our purpose by keeping us focused on shrinking our bodies.

Let's Define Diet Culture

In her book *Anti-Diet: Reclaim Your Time, Money, Well-Being, and Happiness through Intuitive Eating,* Christy Harrison, a registered dietitian and colleague, defines diet culture as "a system of beliefs that equates thinness, muscularity, and particular body shapes with health and moral virtue; promotes weight loss and body reshaping as a means of attaining higher status, and demonizes certain foods and food groups while elevating others; and oppresses people who don't match its supposed picture of 'health.'"[1] This belief system runs deep in our culture and has historical ties to racism and evangelical legalism around presenting oneself as a pure and worthy Christian (particularly in regard to Christian women). Sabrina Strings, PhD, a professor of sociology and author of *Fearing the Black Body: The Racial Origins of Fat Phobia,* takes an even deeper dive, revealing how racism and classism have shaped our so-called war on ob*sity.[2] It is a worthy read for everyone navigating this culture.

We need all the reminders we can get in this culture. So you'll hear me say this many times throughout this book: body diversity is divine. The "one size fits all" body type isn't real, and it's harmful, particularly if it's the church that is perpetuating this notion. We, the church's people, must dismantle this system within our walls. But first we must be able to see it.

Now, you may be thinking that dieting and maintaining a "healthy weight" make you a "healthy" Christian by being a good steward of your body. It makes perfect sense to feel that way because diet culture is often the lens through which we read the Bible and also influences scientific research, medical recommendations, and education. Many books by well-known Christian authors urge readers to follow weight-loss diets, use privileged grocery lists, abstain from sugar, or merely pray over their next diet. Again, I'm sure these leaders had the best intentions, but harm can still be the result. Wrapping a diet, detox, or meal plan in Bible verses doesn't make it truth; it makes it dangerous, and the enemy loves it.

Just as the offhand comments about dieting overheard at church functions are deeply rooted in diet culture, so too are our community health policies. According to Business Wire, the U.S. diet industry is worth more than $70 billion.[3] When I say diet culture, you may be thinking about WW (formerly Weight Watchers), Jenny Craig, Atkins, Noom, Keto, and calorie-tracking apps, but it's so much bigger. We see diet culture in the dizzying array of supplements and shakes on the market. We see it in the exercise programs that promise weight loss and in the "you can look like me" influencers. Diet culture is even in our everyday conversations among friends—"That burger looks so good, but I should really order the salad." It's everywhere.

Diet culture is entangled in industry studies, research funding, and scientific conclusions. Many of the scientists and professionals involved with medical and health policy also have financial ties to the weight-loss industry. These egregiously biased studies have become the foundation for medical, public health, and educational guidelines. Emerging evidence calls out this bias and points to the need for reform in health and weight policy.[4]

It's in All the "Safe" Places

Sometimes when I give examples of diet culture in the church, people aren't sure what I mean because the teachings are so often wrapped up, falsely, as " health" messages. A well-meaning preacher may teach that nothing can separate us from the love of Christ and then turn around and say, "But let's talk about your health." Diet culture is insidious—it's a sneaky chameleon. So it just seems normal when diet culture messages slip into church sermons, small group chatter, and Bible studies. And that's just the tip of the iceberg when we consider how diet culture shows up in the church. We'll dig deeper in later chapters.

The lies of diet culture are around every corner. When my daughter was about two years old, I can clearly remember a villainous pack of french fries chasing a pure and perfect apple superhero on a little kids television channel. That was followed by "get your body back" messages for moms. I've read body- and food-shaming passages in elementary language arts lessons, and I've seen a Thanksgiving math packet that included counting calories and suggested making "good" or "bad" decisions based on the sums. A family friend may scold a parent and child for the child's (very normal) prepubescent weight gain and recommend a diet. These are all incredibly harmful messages to which we've grown accustomed. It's simply an everyday expectation, like seeing weight-loss tips on magazine covers at the grocery checkout. And we can be sure that little eyes see those too.

I'm not saying we shouldn't pursue health in a way that feels

WHERE CAN WE FIND DIET CULTURE?

Diet culture is the rule, not the exception. Consequently, it can be hard to see, even in places we think are safe. Here are some examples of how diet culture is manifested and why these messages are wrong.

Medical Offices— Children	Encouraging children and parents to "do something" about normal weight changes. *Growth equates to weight gain.*
Medical Offices— Adults	Starting an office visit by stepping on the scale. *Weight checks are, for the most part, unnecessary for adult medical visits.*
Churches— Children	Allowing only "healthy" snacks at Sunday school. *There is no "one size fits all" definition of health or healthy food.*
Churches— Adults	Hearing comments such as, "Oh, I shouldn't be eating this," or "Why do they always have so many sweets at fellowship events?" *Worrying about food ingredients is far worse for us than eating a cupcake.*
Schools— Elementary	Assigning homework that asks children to categorize food into "good" or "bad." *Dichotomizing food creates food and body distrust and often causes the child to feel like they're bad for wanting or eating those foods.*
Schools— Secondary	Making assignments such as calorie-counting records and discussing "healthy" weights. *Focusing on numbers creates a deep disconnect within our bodies so that we don't understand our own hunger and fullness signals. This kind of focus also disconnects us from our food, which becomes nothing more than numbers, whether it's calories, macros, or sugar grams.*
Media— Radio	A Christian radio station talks about "clean" eating and how calories from Christmas cookies don't count. *Calorie counting and labeled ways of eating aren't necessary for divinely created bodies.*
Media— Social	Prominent Christian influencers suggest sugar fasts or praying over "unhealthy" food choices. *The fear of making "good" choices comes from diet culture, not from an all-powerful God.*

right to us. I'm saying we don't need diet culture to define our health and well-being for us. We'll touch much more on defining health for you and your own family in later chapters. But as Jesus followers, we must be aware of the dangers of diet culture in our congregations, our schools, and the places where we receive medical advice. When we're engaging in it, diet culture negatively influences our physical, mental, and spiritual wellness. It is the thief of calling. It is the thief of purpose. It will steal the glory of God that is to be lived out through us, whether we realize it or not.

As the lies of diet culture settle into our belief systems, this philosophy can become the primary lens through which we see the world. We may read Bible verses about the body and eating and automatically think we are called to change our bodies or eat less. We may look for diets to help us feel more accepted in this world, though we are *already* known and loved by God. We may even get wrapped up in social groups that have one thing in common—supporting each other on the weight-loss journey, no matter what it takes. Before we know it, we're living for the blessing of strangers who are also immersed in diet culture. We can quickly find that our mental health and physical health are degraded, and we become obsessed with a no-excuses mindset, leaving no room for celebrating divine body diversity or reveling in God's grace.

The negative influence of diet culture takes our time and attention away from using the gifts God has given us. It is so hard to use our spiritual gifts when we're not fed. We can't think. We can't serve. We begin to serve macros and calories and the scale, forfeiting our gifts that bring glory to God. This isn't our fault. But diet culture isn't going anywhere anytime soon. And it's getting sneakier and sneakier at making us think *we* are the problem.

Diet Culture Will Always Make Us Feel like We're Not Good Enough

Companies profit from our insecurities through trying to sell us the cure. Diet culture is found anywhere anything is sold or taught and takes various forms—clothing, devotionals, books, social media, food, fitness, toys, medicine, and academics. Take, for example, my education and training as a registered dietitian/nutritionist. Sadly, when studying nutrition and dietetics in college, I began to overthink the foods I ate and their lists of ingredients. Looking back, I realized that what I was learning in my nutrition program was riddled with diet culture lessons that lacked unbiased nutritional science and feeding development research. Many interns and students I meet today have little or no training in honoring our uniquely designed bodies as a true path toward wellness. No wonder we feel so torn! It can feel like we may never get it right.

You've likely gone through a season when you overscrutinized what you ate, given the pervasive influence of our diet-obsessed culture. You may still be in a season of suffering when it comes to your relationship with food and your body. If that's the case, you don't have to remain stuck. And please don't beat yourself up over it, even if you're a pastor, ministry leader, Christian influencer, or healthcare professional. We can't swim in the waters of this culture and not get wet. It is everywhere, but we can learn to swim upstream.

Believers must begin to see diet culture for what it is—a deceptive tool of the enemy that must be recognized by everyone, especially faith leaders, and denounced in the church. If the enemy can keep a whole church participating in a diet program together instead of fueling their divine vessels, it makes for deeply distracted and, quite frankly, not very useful followers. An underfed believer is easy prey.

When we're weight-obsessed and running on fumes, we have little energy left to fight oppression, seek mercy and justice, live out our purpose, and accept God's marvelous grace.

I recently listened to a past episode of the *Dream Big Podcast* with Bob Goff and Friends in which he chatted with bestselling Christian author and well-known preacher Max Lucado about engaging the world with hope. Goff said something that made me rewind the words over and over: "If we want to do something just glorious for Jesus, why don't we start by being who we are."[5] It clutched my heart and sealed this message about the way diet culture steals the very essence of us, our potential, and our acceptance of these divine vessels.

> When we're **weight-obsessed** and running on fumes, we have little energy left to fight oppression, seek mercy and justice, live out our purpose, and accept God's marvelous grace.

As we start to see diet culture for what it is—a thief of joy and purpose— let's be who we are! I pray that all of us can one day feel safe to celebrate who we were created to be, no matter our body's shape or size. I do want to acknowledge that it's easier for me to say this—since I live in a body that hasn't been marginalized or discriminated against. We can work together to help make this world safer for *all bodies* by recognizing that we all play a role in supporting and celebrating body diversity. In doing so, I hope we can remember that we are all fearfully and wonderfully made by a God who is bigger than our culture, bigger even than our perceptions of health. God isn't interested in a number on a scale or the size of our jeans. God cares about the state of our hearts.

THE WORLD SAYS . . .

If you control your body by manipulating the food you eat and the way your body looks, you will achieve health and be more valuable.

THE WORD SAYS . . .

The thief comes only to steal and kill and destroy; I have come that they may have life, and have it to the full.

John 10:10

STEPPING AWAY FROM LIES

Think about how diet culture surrounds us and permeates almost every aspect of our lives.

- Do you have early memories of how diet culture showed up in your life? It may have been in lessons taught at school or comments from a trusted teacher or counselor.

- Did you witness diet culture in your church? Do you see it in your social circle or your church groups?

- Can you see how diet culture creates an earthly hierarchy of bodies (definitely not from God)? When we learn in this culture that some bodies are more valuable than others, how can we realize this message isn't from God?

- Review John 10:10. If you're like most people in this culture (including me), can you see how diet culture has stolen time and other things from your life? What has it stolen?

- Can you see how diet culture harms people who have bodies that don't align with the cultural value of thinness? How will you continue to detect diet culture?

It's Simple! Calories In, Calories Out

> I did then what I knew how to do. Now that I know better, I do better.
>
> **Maya Angelou**

I posted a story on social media that got more attention than my usual posts. It read, "If you are a health or fitness professional who recommends intentional weight loss and dieting, please understand that you are also promoting intentional disordered eating." Many readers commented on how they had come to discover the harm in calorie counting or mentioned how dismissed they felt when a medical professional recommended weight loss after they'd come in for something as simple as a flu shot. Some even suggested that the health professional's unsolicited calorie-counting and weight-loss advice opened the door to their eating disorder.

One well-meaning fitness professional agreed that people

shouldn't diet and suggested a "calories in, calories out" approach instead. Because diet culture can put a pretend health spin on any trend, he just didn't realize that "calories in, calories out" is intentional weight loss and dieting. No matter how you spin it, calorie math *is* dieting, and it has been the most common way to diet for decades. It's not new or different. It has simply been repackaged over and over, decade after decade. In all my years as an eating disorder dietitian, the "calories in, calories out" mindset has been the slippery slope into deprivation for almost every one of my clients.

No matter how you spin it, calorie math *is* dieting.

I had to fail my way to this knowledge as well. Early in my career as a dietitian, I counted my calories. It was a reprieve from the fat-gram book I'd had in college. Before apps came along, we had web-based programs we could log on to each day to record each food we had at a meal. I'd keep up with the meals and snacks, hoping to keep my total intake under a certain amount each day. I thought that was just what "good" dietitians did. Practice what you preach, right? In those early years, I stuck close to the nutrition program's numbers we focused on so keenly. The majority of the "nutrition" I learned about and studied was more about seeing how little of it you could get. Not very nutritious, huh?

That was more than two decades ago. And let me tell you, I am so grateful for the unlearning I've had the privilege to engage in since then. This unlearning and subsequent relearning came early in my career when I realized that calorie counting wasn't bringing health or wellness to me or my patients. Rather, this approach brought me anxiety and strife with regard to food and food planning, not to mention my body. It reminded me of the dieting habits I watched so many people engage in as I was growing up. It seemed wrong even then, but it was what I knew.

Growing up, I picked up on two main factors when it came to diet: fat is evil, and getting rid of fat will lower the calories. And that should make it "healthy." The numbers I learned in school seemed to fall right in line with what I had absorbed in my youth. It seemed like nutrition was all about the numbers or the sexier "point system." If you committed to this system, the numbers would lead you to health (a.k.a. thinness). Well, nothing could be further from the truth.

Imagine a time when there were no food labels, no apps for tracking every morsel, and no nutrient databases. Humans thrived long before we relied on these numbers to guide us. For thousands of years, members of the human race fed themselves without external oversight or controls.

The Birth of the Nutrition Facts Label

Before the 1960s, little to no information was available on food packaging. Over the years, laws and regulations around labeling for specific ingredients, nutrient content, and marketing claims became more mainstream. In 1990, the Nutrition Labeling and Education Act was passed into law, making it mandatory for most food packaging to contain nutrition information.[1] And so in the early 1990s, the Nutrition Facts label as we know it was born. Before then, humans were able to eat and make decisions about eating without all the information and numbers.

Over the next two decades, not much changed on the labels—until 2020, when the Nutrition Facts label got an update. According to the U.S. Food and Drug Administration, these label changes make it "easier for consumers to make better informed food choices."[2] Guess what was the most prominent change on the label? Yep! The size and font of the number of calories. I can tell you in the highest confidence that on the rare occasion when I talk about food labels in my office to help people make informed food choices, we are *not* focusing on calories.

NUTRITION FACTS LABELS

Nutrition Facts label alterations and additions that are crucial for the health and safety of some consumers have been made along the way, like the "Ingredients" and "Contains" lists (e.g., eggs, tree nuts, shellfish). This label information can be important for those with certain health conditions or medically diagnosed food allergies. Information about carbohydrates can help those who use insulin dose their medicine. There are times when information about production location and manufacturing practices can help isolate foods that have been recalled. While the label is helpful at times for some people, we tend to put the most focus on certain items on the label, such as calories, serving size, and diet culture "health" claims, when in reality these items often matter the least.

It makes sense that we're obsessed with calories. The Nutrition Facts label has perpetuated for decades the misconception that calories are one of the most critical factors in health—even though the calculations, which are actually estimates, are allowed *to be wrong*. In fact, the law allows the estimates to be off by as much as 20 percent.[3] We've assumed for a long time that we can count on this information to be accurate. Not only might the calorie numbers be inaccurate, but they also can't account for physiological differences from person to person. Our digestive systems are not controlled science labs.

A tremendous amount of variability exists in the nutrient and energy extraction from food from person to person, as well as in food processing and cooking methods. For instance, the digestion, absorption, and metabolizable energy of protein, fat, and carbohydrates can depend on the nutrient mix of a meal, an individual's microbiome, and even the way foods are chewed.[4] Because of these variances, the calorie number on a food package isn't necessarily the amount of energy your body will get from that food. It is by no means as simple as a number on a food label.

These energy values, or caloric numbers used as the basis for estimating the numbers on the Nutrition Fact labels, were flawed from the start. Additionally, Wilbur Atwater, the scientist responsible for creating the system that measures the metabolizable energy provided by food—calories—we use for food labeling today, stated that he had made many assumptions and poor decisions in his experiments.[5] Yet more than a century later, we rely on this information for labeling and, subsequently, making many health-based decisions.

We've built decades of diet programs on shaky numbers and bogus claims that this math will solve our ills. We have falsely assumed that a "calories in, calories out" approach is the way to health via weight control. However, studies suggest energy regulation and body size aren't that simple; they involve a complex dance between the body's needs, genetics, and environment and our endocrine, metabolic, and nervous systems.[6] We are diversely and intricately made.

Our health systems, which are sadly often a part of the diet industrial complex, have also perpetuated the notion that our wellness boils down to simple math. And because we have so much trust in our health and medical systems, this thinking has trickled down into schools, homes, and churches. Please don't assume it's our fault. We've been sold a false bill of goods. But now it is our job to see the lie. This "calories in, calories out," pretend health equation is untrue and dangerous.

What Did All This Calorie Counting Get Us?

The short answer is this: it got us an epidemic of humans struggling with disordered eating. It's no wonder—the food tracker tells us we need x number of calories; the health article in the rack at the checkout lane says this many calories. Now, humor me . . . Which one is the right choice? Most of us would think it's the lowest one because we've been programmed in diet culture to think less is more. It's untrue. *Neither* option is good for us.

Less is simply less. Less food equals less life. Less calories means less mental capacity to connect with the humans around us. Ultimately, less energy equals falling down the rabbit hole of a starved life. Diet culture has sanctioned our collective starvation—often with a well-meaning health professional's stamp of approval.

I am very cautious when stating or discussing numbers like calories and weight because I know it can be triggering for people. Only on rare occasions will I share calorie numbers specifically because it can keep people stuck relying on external controls when it comes to eating. However, in this instance I think they're worth noting because these are the calorie levels we see casually recommended today on health and fitness apps, in magazines, and even by some health professionals.

I had this kind of conversation with Nicole, whom you met in the introduction. Nicole had been counting calories for years. The app she used recommended energy levels that would not support her body's basic needs, not to mention the increased energy needs of her job, exercise regimen, and care for her kids. She was starving and blaming herself for feeling hungry and "out of control" with food. These numbers may seem normal and appropriate, but they're not.

It's common today to see recommended calorie levels that are lower than the calorie levels of the landmark starvation studies of the late 1940s. During the Second World War, Ancel Keys, a professor at the University of Minnesota, was curious about how the civilians who had endured the German occupation lived on so little nourishment.[7] Very little was known about how starvation affected the human body. Keys recruited thirty-six conscientious objectors—healthy men who refused to go to war because they believed it was wrong to take another human life. They wanted to help their country—but not through war.

The study's participants began with a daily intake of about 3,200 calories for about three months, and subsequently their daily intake decreased to about 1,800 calories for the next six months.[8] During that semi-starvation period, they were also asked to exercise and burn off calories. The participants' starvation led to obsessive thoughts about food, a compulsion to sneak food, and mental health decline. They also experienced dizziness, edema, hair loss, poor concentration, loss of sex drive, fatigue, and a continual chill in their bodies.[9] Once this period was over, even a daily intake of 2,000 calories couldn't rehabilitate them. They needed far more energy—almost double that amount—to heal from the starvation period.[10]

I surely don't want us counting or stressing over calories. But when I talk about these numbers, it is for one reason only—to make the point that we need far more than we've been taught in diet culture. Nicole couldn't get over how similar her experience with dieting was to the experience of those who had volunteered to starve. She faced many of the same side effects reported by the study's participants. Nicole thought her calorie restriction would be good for her, and even her friends and family supported her. But ultimately her mental and physical health suffered. We've forgotten, and often ignored, this historical experiment. The result? Many of us are slowly and quite possibly starving in diet culture.

Many of us are slowly and quite possibly starving in diet culture.

Much of the time, disordered eating behaviors and eating disorders are built on a foundation of calorie counting. Research suggests that calorie and fitness tracking is associated with eating disorder symptoms.[11] This association has been true in my experience in my office as well. The fact that the incidence of eating disorders has more than doubled worldwide in the last twenty years comes as no surprise.[12] Our culture has endorsed it. Demonizing calories—those little units of life-giving energy—may have paved the way for this mind-boggling increase.

It Doesn't Have to Continue

When we see the truth, it's hard to unsee it and return to the lie. We are all *fearfully and wonderfully made*—every single human being. I believe this with all my heart. We are in direct conflict with this belief when we count calories, obsess over macros, live by a "righteous" grocery list, or purposely try to reduce or conform our bodies to a cultural ideal. We are far more glorious—and complex—than simple math.

THE WORLD SAYS . . .

You must micromanage every bite and calorie, and only then will you be worthy and "healthy."

THE WORD SAYS . . .

Do not set your heart on what you will eat or drink; do not worry about it.

Luke 12:29

STEPPING AWAY FROM LIES

Calories are not heavenly currency. The
Bible makes no mention of counting the
food we consume. Diet culture is the reason
we are so determined to count calories.

- Could calorie counting be distracting us from
  doing God's work?

- How does it make you feel to know the numbers
  can be wrong?

- If you're a calorie counter (and it makes sense
  that you might be) and you decide to let those
  numbers go, what could you do with the time and
  focus you got back?

- Can you think of calories, or the little units of
  energy they are, as life-giving gifts from an all-
  powerful God? Can you see them as a means to
  live out your purpose?

- Think about Luke 12:29. How can you begin to
  look at this verse with a fresh and fed vision?

Health Equals Diet and Exercise

> Anyone who gets to the end of their life with the exact same beliefs and opinions as they had at the beginning is doing it wrong.
>
> **Sarah Bessey, *Out of Sorts***

We've learned to believe our health hangs in the balance according to what we eat and how much we exercise. It is diet culture that profits from this false belief, not those who seek the truth. The "just get your diet and exercise in check" approach to health is incredibly shortsighted. It ignores lived experience in this world and leaves us languishing. Let me tell you about Edward.

Edward reached out to see if I could help him make some nutritional changes. He had been suffering from digestive issues and sleep disturbances for quite a while. Over the past months, he had gone to doctor after doctor. The recommendations kept circling back to his diet, even though not one of these professionals asked him about what he regularly ate, what his stress level was like, or what his day-to-day schedule looked like. Time after time, he got the typical cookie-cutter approach to all things health—*change your diet.*

In our first session, we reviewed his concerns and dove into his beliefs around food, movement, and health. He'd been an active person all his life. He felt like his symptoms didn't add up. He had done what he thought was necessary to maintain the "standard" views of health. Edward didn't realize that his body was experiencing symptoms most likely unrelated to his diet or exercise.

During our time together, he shared more about his daily schedule and his volatile work environment. Every single day he worked in dangerous conditions. He was fully aware of what he'd be facing when he signed up for this occupation. He felt like this job was his calling, but that sense of purpose didn't make it easier for him.

Edward had experienced trauma after trauma. His body was responding the only way it could—survival mode. Though he likely wasn't eating enough to carry out the work of healing, his symptoms weren't caused by his food intake or exercise; they were the manifestation of a traumatized nervous system constantly on high alert. Food can't fix what the body isn't meant to endure.

WHAT IS HEALTH?

The World Health Organization (WHO) defines health as "a state of complete physical, mental and social well-being and not merely the absence of disease or infirmity."[1] As you can see, health is much more than diet and exercise.

Diet and Exercise Are Only a Small Part of What Contributes to Health

Health isn't the sum of food on a plate and time on a treadmill. The solutions to a complex life can't be whittled down to diet and exercise. That's a lie of diet culture. Sometimes there are no solutions. Sometimes medication or another medical intervention is required. Sometimes health depends on lowering our stress levels. Health is multifaceted, and contrary to our culture's "conventional wisdom," it looks different for everyone.

Most of us are trained to think that health results mainly from our behaviors. I used to believe that my health status was good because I had made many "right" choices throughout life. After all, I was taught that health is simple mix of eating a "good" diet, getting plenty of exercise, and refraining from smoking. But this was an ill-informed view. Health is a complicated web of not just genetics and privileges but environmental and social factors as well.

> Health is multifaceted, and contrary to our culture's **"conventional wisdom,"** it looks different for everyone.

PRIVILEGE

Let's talk about *privilege*. Just hearing this word can ruffle feathers, but we're going to address it anyway because it matters. If it bothers you, stick with me. It used to bother me too—until I learned more about what it meant.

For some people, the word feels like an attack on their work ethic. They may think, *I worked hard for x, y, or z, which is why I have what I have in life.* It may also look like a priority issue; for example, *If so-and-so cared more about their health, they would do a, b, or c or buy x, y, or z.* But that's not really what it's all about. I used to think like this until I allowed myself to see privilege as being more of a *benefit*, which is part of the actual definition. The internet defines privilege as "a particular benefit, advantage, or favor; a right or immunity enjoyed by some but not others."[2]

While practicing unlearning and relearning, I've come to acknowledge my privileges. The "work hard" and "set better priorities" arguments suggest that many individuals may not be aware of the very different lived experiences of others and the way their experiences influence the choices they make. Here are a few examples of privileges that are often unacknowledged:

- Having access to non-stigmatizing medical care (that is, you didn't get a weight lecture or diet recommendation for having pink eye or a cold).
- Living near a grocery store and being able to afford enough food for you and your family (that is, you can easily get to a variety of food stores and don't have to decide between buying food and paying bills).
- Being able to go out for a walk in your neighborhood and feel safe (that is, you have access to sidewalks, live in a safe neighborhood, and are able-bodied).

Recognizing privilege doesn't mean we haven't worked hard; it simply means we understand that other people can work just as hard and still not have the same benefits. This insight has allowed me to understand better how someone's lived experience can have an influence on their decisions—decisions that may look very different from mine. This acknowledgment has allowed me to grow in compassion and care for others. I invite you to reflect on your own benefits.

According to the Centers for Disease Control and Prevention (CDC), the definition of social determinants of health (SDOH) are "conditions in the places where people live, learn, work, and play that affect a wide range of health risks and outcomes."[3] The World Health Organization defines the SDOH as the "non-medical factors that influence health outcomes. They are the conditions in which people are born, grow, work, live, and age, and the wider set of forces and systems shaping the conditions of daily life. These forces and systems include economic policies and systems, development agendas, social norms, social policies, and political systems."[4]

I wish I had gained a strong understanding of the social determinants of health (SDOH) in my undergraduate and graduate degree programs. Knowing these determinants should be a crucial area of study for all medical and health degree programs. When we miss out on this foundational piece of education, we may overlook underlying issues that cause health concerns, making it possible our practice will be based on assumptions about someone's life or health choices and not on thorough evaluation and assessment.

Healthism, a lifestyle that puts the pursuit of health and fitness over everything else, has become its own religion.

It makes sense to focus on diet and exercise. Healthism, a lifestyle that puts the pursuit of health and fitness over everything else, has become its own religion. But diet and exercise are the whipped cream and sprinkles on top of the ice cream sundae. We're failing to address the foundation. One of the largest scoops on which all the other toppings fall consists of the SDOH. We've focused on diet and exercise because the whipped cream and sprinkles are easier to swallow. Blaming an individual if they're perceived as "unhealthy" is a faster and tidier way to move along the "care" process than acknowledging long-standing systems of oppression.

According to the World Health Organization, health and illness tend to follow a social gradient. Regardless of the income of the country, those in lower socioeconomic positions will suffer from poorer health.[5] Health is clearly determined by more than diet and exercise. The social determinants of health may pave the road to health possibilities or disparities, but the experience of trauma also plays a dramatic role in our health and well-being.

SOCIAL DETERMINANTS OF HEALTH

The U.S. Department of Health and Human Services defines the social determinants of health as "the conditions in the environments where people are born, live, learn, work, play, worship, and age that affect a wide range of health, functioning, and quality-of-life outcomes and risks."[6]

When I learned about the social determinants of health, the puzzle pieces didn't suddenly snap into place. The box of pieces exploded, showing me that individual health is profoundly more complicated and multifaceted than I was ever taught or realized. It was eye-opening. It's important to recognize we all start with different foundational elements or pieces. Here are a few examples of SDOH that can impact health over our life spans:

- prenatal care
- early childhood development care
- timely medical screenings
- non-stigmatizing healthcare
- safe and consistent housing
- reliable transportation
- education and literacy skills
- solid employment status and job security
- safe job conditions
- clean air and water
- food security
- freedom from racism, discrimination, violence, and generational trauma

> Child abuse and neglect is the single most preventable cause of **mental illness,** the single most common cause of drug and alcohol abuse, and a significant contributor to leading causes of death such as diabetes, heart disease, cancer, stroke, and suicide.
>
> Bessel A. van der Kolk,
> *The Body Keeps the Score*

Take a moment to think about your social determinants of health. You may be among the fortunate who have experienced little negative impact. You may have dealt with food insecurity or had inadequate access to non-stigmatizing medical care.[7] You may have been discriminated against in healthcare or educational settings.

Have You Heard of Adverse Childhood Events (ACEs)?

I hadn't heard of "adverse childhood events" until a few years ago. Mark this as another area of study that all health, medical, and mental health practitioners should undertake before seeing patients in the professional world. ACEs are situations or events that harm children or adolescents through either neglect or abuse. Not everyone experiences ACEs, but many adults have experienced one or more of these events during their childhood. When I learned about ACEs, I thought of many of my clients who had suffered in this way and how those experiences had affected their health.

ACEs increase the risk of adverse health concerns over a person's life span. These events include childhood exposure to violence, abuse, neglect, untreated mental health issues, substance abuse, and caregiver imprisonment. It's estimated that nearly 61 percent of American adults have suffered at least one ACE exposure, and almost 15 percent have four or more ACEs.[8] The more ACEs a person has, the greater the likelihood they'll experience health problems such as heart disease, cancer, chronic lung disease, skeletal fractures, and liver disease later in life.[9] You may be thinking what I'm thinking: *So many of these conditions are blamed on diet and exercise.* And that is true. We've got work to do.

ADVERSE CHILDHOOD EXPERIENCES

If you're interested in learning more about adverse childhood experiences, you can read more on the CDC's website.[10] Knowing more about ACEs can help us understand ourselves and our neighbors a little better. If you decide to examine your own ACEs score (what it means and doesn't mean), please reach out to a trauma-informed medical or mental health professional to discuss your results.

Traumas experienced in adulthood also impact our physical and mental wellness, such as in the situation Edward experienced (see his story at the beginning of this chapter). I'm not suggesting that every person with health concerns has experienced trauma—that's simply not the case. But many people have endured the fear of food insecurity and the absence of a stable home. Others have experienced childhood or adult traumas and have been given the tools to work through those wounds so they carry less hurt over time. What I'm saying is that we can't ignore the evidence that leads us to conclude that SDOH, ACEs, and trauma play a huge role in our health. Acknowledging that there's more to health than diet and exercise may just lead us to a more genuine healing.

We must care more about lifelong well-being than the illusion of health control through diet and exercise. It's time to put to rest the old "pull yourself up by your bootstraps" way of thinking. This assumption that everyone can achieve health and other things through their own willpower and hard work is incredibly shortsighted. Once upon a time, I used to think that way. But a very wise man named Martin Luther King Jr. taught us that not everyone has boots: "It's a cruel jest to say to a bootless man that he ought to lift himself up by his own bootstraps."[11] You can't pull up or put on something you've never had. It's a cruel expectation.

It's time for a new way of thinking that offers compassion and grace to all of our neighbors. We have no idea what others have been through or are going through in this world. I pray that God helps us remember it's not our job to judge or make assumptions; rather, our job is to love and care for others, as well as ourselves.

THE WORLD SAYS . . .

Your health is ultimately up to you. Get your
diet and exercise in check if you want to
be healthy, happy, loved, and worthy.

THE WORD SAYS . . .

I am convinced that nothing can ever separate us
from God's love. Neither death nor life, neither
angels nor demons, neither our fears for today
nor our worries about tomorrow—not even the
powers of hell can separate us from God's love.

Romans 8:38 NLT

STEPPING AWAY FROM LIES

I'm asking you to rethink your belief
system around health, and I know how
hard it is to do so. I've done it myself.

- Do you need to broaden your view of health? For yourself? For others?

- If you do expand your view, what areas of health will you now acknowledge that you hadn't realized before?

- Have you experienced ACEs or traumatic events as an adult? You are not alone.

- Did you realize that the social determinants of heath have such a significant influence on the foundation of health? Think about these factors as we continue on in the chapters ahead. There's so much more to come.

- Take a moment to reflect on Romans 8:38. Hear the truth expressed there: *nothing* can separate us from God's love—not even an earthly view or expectation of health.

It's Not a Diet—
It's a Lifestyle

> Nothing that's truly healthy for you will require you to step out of your character, belittle your standards, mistreat yourself, or shrink your voice and existence to keep it. Absolutely nothing. No space, relationship, or opportunity is worth that much peace.
>
> **Terence Lester, Twitter post, March 3, 2022, 8:24 a.m.**

It's my job to help you see diet culture. That's what I tell my clients. Once we start to see it all around us, we can't unsee it. We may even have some righteous anger around diet culture and how it has lied to us, our families, and our friends. We can become better equipped to fight the good fight when we know what we're up against.

One of the most common ways diet culture disguises itself is through a phrase I used to say often: "It's not a diet—it's a lifestyle." I hate to admit it, but I did. And you had better believe I stood by it. I'd give you a meal plan and spout a version of this "balanced way of eating for life, not a diet plan" philosophy. At that time, the meal plans were very much a diet, akin to the more recent and sexier "macro-counting lifestyle" plans. Looking back now, I can see it. I wasn't helping people implement health behaviors that would be sustainable throughout their life spans; I was peddling diet culture. I was arrogant. I was naive. I was trying to help. I was dishing out what people said they wanted, not knowing it was harmful.

Luckily, not long after my "diet culture sold here" days, a group of lovely therapists took me under their wings. They taught me about eating disorders and intuitive eating. They took me to conferences that helped me understand family dynamics and dysfunction. They taught me about mental health disorders and trauma. They led me into a state of cognitive dissonance, a feeling of being pulled away from what I learned in school and life toward a completely different way of helping and healing.

Because diet culture is sneaky, it can take us off-road, even when we think we have the best guardrails.

I found myself torn between what I'd been taught in life and in higher education and an approach that leaves the numbers behind. I started trying to find ways to see and support a whole person and their lived experience. It took a couple of years of unlearning and relearning, but I finally stepped away from the dark side (a.k.a. diet culture). And I'm committed to continuing my learning. Because diet culture is sneaky, it can take us off-road, even when we think we have the best guardrails.

Holly Had Sturdy Guardrails

As a teen, Holly battled an eating disorder. She was lucky enough to have a complete treatment team of eating disorder–informed health practitioners—a therapist, a dietitian, and a physician. By the time she graduated from high school, she was in recovery and free from the bondage of her disorder. Her guardrails were strong.

Holly made it through college without falling into patterns of disordered eating. A few months after graduating, she landed her first real job. She was super-excited to make her own money, live in her own place and make it a home, and start adulting.

Things were going well at first, but Holly found herself starting to track her food on an app a few months after starting her new job. Like others in her office, she thought it was just one of the many health behaviors she could engage in as an adult without the risk of falling back into disordered eating—and she did, until eating less and less became the goal.

When her coworkers started intermittent fasting, Holly concluded that practice needed to be the next step in her healthy lifestyle. After all, she had heard that health professionals recommended it, so how could it be wrong? However, it did turn out to be wrong. All of the tracking and restriction dressed up as a healthy lifestyle led her to circle the drain of disordered eating again.

The intermittent fasting lifestyle trend flipped the switch that led her straight back to her eating disorder. We don't even need to have a history of disordered eating or an eating disorder for this to happen. Research suggests that those who adopt an intermittent fasting approach have significantly higher scores on eating disorder questionnaires and are more likely to have eating disorder symptoms.[1] It's just another diet dressed up as a "healthy lifestyle."

We All Know "Diets Don't Work"

I bet you've heard over and over for years that diets don't work to improve our health; on the contrary, they make us sick, tired, and hangry. But diets do work . . . *for the diet industry.* Selling diet plans pads their wallets with billions of dollars, not to make us well, but to compel us to return over and over with each failed attempt. If diets worked, WW wouldn't offer a lifetime membership. But we keep coming back because diets do work in the short term, and we've been tricked into thinking it's us and not them when the weight returns. But our bodies aren't meant to starve—that's what diet culture doesn't want us to figure out.

Diet culture corners the market on predatory marketing, which is why "It's not a diet—it's a lifestyle" is the New Age slogan. Same crappy diet, shiny new bow—the same ol' wolf in sheep's clothing. We fall victim to it because the "not a diet diet" marketing is so alluring and is often backed by health professionals. Evidence exists to warn us of the harm of dieting—warnings that are chronically and purposefully ignored, even by professional health organizations.

When evidence of harm is ignored, the status quo can continue. There are no demands to change practices, philosophies, or programs, and diet culture is empowered to change its look into a "lifestyle" or "wellness" program such as Wellness Works (WW, formerly Weight Watchers), Noom (a super-sneaky "not a diet diet" like WW), keto (the "malnourished constipation" diet), intermittent fasting (the "starve all day, binge later" diet), Optivia (the expensive "malnutrition with community support" diet), and so many more. By the time this book is in your hands, dozens more will be added to the list.

If a "lifestyle" or wellness program compels you to outsource your God-given inner wisdom to a points system, macro counter, calorie calculator, stoplight colors, or food coach, I assure you that diet culture is behind the wheel. It may feel great at first (the diet culture hook), but over and over, it causes us harm instead of helps us. That's the trap. Diet culture knows how to steal the language of sound health-behavior research and even eating disorder treatment philosophies so we keep coming back. When the programs fail, and they *will* fail, we don't hate them; we hate *ourselves*.

> If a "lifestyle" or wellness program compels you to outsource your God-given **inner wisdom** to a points system, macro counter, calorie calculator, stoplight colors, or food coach, I assure you that diet culture is behind the wheel.

The whole secret of the diet industry is this: none of the diets work, but when they don't work, it's always our fault. We'll question ourselves before we question their motives. *Maybe I didn't restrict myself enough. Maybe I just didn't do it right. I wonder if I don't have enough willpower. I bet if I would've given it another week or two, it would have worked.* Somehow it feels like it's always our fault, and we are quick to accept the blame. After all, diet culture taught us from an early age that we must be faulty or we wouldn't have needed the diet in the first place.

It's possible we'll even find ourselves defending a program that didn't "work" for us. Perhaps we'll advocate for it because of those "good" parts. And it makes sense. We don't want to believe we've invested time, energy, and money in something that failed. Now we're stuck on the hamster wheel of the "not a diet diet" plans. But know this: you did not fail. Diets aren't built to last—even the pretend lifestyle ones.

Get Out of Our Heads, Diet Culture!

If diet culture can keep our minds occupied, think of the talents and dreams it can stifle. These so-called healthy living plans can lead us to dangerous health practices and disordered eating without our even knowing it!

DISORDERED EATING BEHAVIORS

Could you have disordered eating behaviors and not know it? It's very possible. Disordered eating is not rare. A study conducted by the University of North Carolina at Chapel Hill (UNC) and *SELF* magazine suggests that almost 65 percent of American women may have disordered eating behaviors, while a total of 75 percent have negative feelings about food and their bodies. Some of these behaviors may look like:

- chronically attempting to lose weight
- showing extreme distress in response to small weight gains
- cutting out entire food groups
- restricting calories
- skipping meals
- smoking to lose weight

These behaviors may be common and are often endorsed in our culture, but they are not normal or healthy.[2]

Sometimes our drive to achieve a healthy lifestyle can send us down the disordered eating rabbit hole with an unhealthy fixation on being healthy. It can lead to a desire to eat only certain types of food that we deem clean or pure and usually involves a strong sense of righteousness or superiority around our eating practices. This is called orthorexia nervosa. When people suffer from orthorexia, they may be extremely distressed when their allowed foods are not available. They may also spend hours thinking about food and planning their food or have an extreme interest in other people's food choices.[3]

When diets are peddled as simply the latest "healthy lifestyle," we are being doubly duped because it's impossible to have complete control over our health simply through our diet. That's a fantasy invented by diet culture, and we'll talk more about it later. Just remember, a diet as a sure path to health creates a false sense of control over our bodies. So many other things affect our health—genetics, environment, privilege, stress—and it's foolish to believe we can be totally "healthy" simply by controlling what we eat.

> It's impossible to have **complete control** over our health simply through our diet.

Our diet- and health-obsessed culture has indeed taken us down a dangerous path—one that is more common than we may have realized—but there is hope. We can walk away and live well despite diet culture. When one of my clients had full recovery from disordered eating in her grasp, she told me, "After all those years of being trapped in that cage, I finally realized there was no lock on the door." There is no lock on this cage. Let's open the door and walk out together.

THE WORLD SAYS . . .

Try this healthy lifestyle approach. It will make you feel better, lose weight, and live your best life.

THE WORD SAYS . . .

I have told you these things, so that in me you may have peace. In this world you will have trouble. But take heart! I have overcome the world.

John 16:33

STEPPING AWAY FROM LIES

- Have you fallen victim to the "lifestyle" diet ruse? We all have. Don't forget that I used to sell it too. It's a tricky scam!

- Are you feeling stirred to move forward in a different way?

- Is the "lifestyle" diet scheme something you'd feel comfortable discussing in your circles? We don't have to overcome on our own.

- Who feels like a safe companion to talk over this issue with? If you're not ready or unsure about whom to confide in, that's okay. Let's continue moving.

- While you've been keeping your eyes open to diet culture, what are some of the sneakiest things you've seen lately?

- Is there a way to protect yourself and those you love from these messages?

- Did you know there is no lock on the cage?

- How can studying John 16:33 be helpful?

Diet Culture Lie #6

Your Weight Is the Most Important Indicator of Your Health

> Patients don't want weight loss out of nowhere. Often they got the idea . . . wait for it . . . from healthcare practitioners. Part of solving the harm that has been done around this is acknowledging that healthcare practitioners (many of whom have been misinformed themselves) have misinformed patients and created patients who think weight loss is the only path to health.
>
> **Ragen Chastain, *Weight and Healthcare***

For years, Jessica went from doctor to doctor to get help for her debilitating fatigue. She had suffered from fatigue off and on since her teen years. She was now twenty-seven. When Jessica sat in my office, she said she thought getting her food habits in check would be the answer. She wanted desperately to feel better in general, but now her fatigue was interfering with her job and her social time with friends.

Jessica and I worked on making sure she was getting adequate energy throughout the day, since she had grown accustomed to skipping meals and snacks on most days. Though we improved her nutrition, making sure she got adequate and consistent nourishment each day, she remained exhausted. I started to delve into her previous medical visits and the advice she received. Each medical professional Jessica visited over the last three years gave her the same recommendation—"*You'll feel better if you lose weight.*"

I had worked closely with Jessica's therapist in the past, which is why she landed in my office. Both Jessica and her therapist knew I was a weight-neutral practitioner, which, in short, means I don't focus on weight; rather, I focus on the person. Jessica lives in a larger body, which increases her risk of experiencing medical weight stigma and poor care. So when she told me this had been her experience, I was saddened but not surprised. The symptoms she'd been experiencing after years of heavy and irregular periods sounded a lot like an iron deficiency to me.

If Jessica had received genuine healthcare instead of weight care, she could have felt better *years* ago. This failure to offer appropriate interventions and further testing (but give weight-loss advice instead) happens more often than I'd like to admit. It happens all the time, every day, in medical offices all over the world. Some patients even die because of the failure to receive proper care. And in my opinion, this is malpractice.

Weight Has Become the Idol of Our Health Policies and Medical System

Medical offices should feel like safe places, but regrettably, weight stigma is one of the main reasons patients avoid them. When the path from the waiting room to the exam room stops at the scale before blood pressure, temperature, or any other measures are taken, often followed by a massive helping of unsolicited weight talk and body shaming, it's no wonder we feel the need to steer clear. Remember the social determinants of health (SDOH)? Access to *non-stigmatizing* healthcare is one of them.

We have to address weight stigma first when we're talking about weight. Weight stigma is the social rejection and devaluing of people who do not conform to expected body weight and shape standards.[1] If you grew up in diet culture, there's a good chance you have weight bias and have witnessed weight stigma. If you're a health professional—particularly a physician, nurse, medical student, or dietitian—there's an even greater chance you have weight bias.[2] Remember the weight-centric training of healthcare professionals? It certainly makes sense that we have this bias, but we had better do something about it or we'll continue to cause harm.

Weight stigma is an act against a person due to their body size. When we harbor harmful beliefs or stereotypes about persons living in larger bodies, such as they're lazy, poorly motivated, or incompetent, our weight bias can turn into actions of weight stigma. Jessica was a victim of weight stigma in healthcare. You may have experienced this as well. When Jessica and I discussed her encounters in greater depth, she said she had come to grips with the bias because she was used to it. But it's *not* okay. It is trauma perpetuated over and over in a supposedly

CHECKING OUR OWN BIAS

We all have a bias. You can't grow up in this culture without having weight bias, but we can and must work on changing our hearts and minds. Here are some examples of weight-biased thinking and untrue assumptions we need to challenge:

- If a person just worked out more or ate less, they could have a "normal" or thin body.
- A person with a larger body must eat more than people with smaller bodies.
- A larger-bodied person must be in poor health.
- People in larger bodies don't care about their health.
- A person with a larger body can't be a fit person.
- People in smaller bodies must be healthier than people in larger bodies.

safe place. We promptly found her a new provider—one who was willing to treat her compassionately, run some simple lab tests, and treat her accordingly, all without focusing on the number on the scale.

Weight is *not* a representation of health. I know, I know— we've been collectively "watching" our weight our entire lives, believing the lie that weight is a deeply significant measure of our health. The public health guidelines that suggest we diet and chase a number on the scale often backfire and cause poorer health.[3] But much of our weight-science research is heavily biased toward thin bodies. Researchers calling for a change in health policy have shown that significant and inaccurate assumptions are made about body size—for example, a higher body weight automatically means a person is unhealthy, diets can promote long-term weight loss, and loss of weight equals better health.[4] In short, many research studies are being carried out to support predetermined hypotheses—such as larger bodies are wrong and therefore must be in poorer health. (I'm married to a researcher, and I can tell you, this is *not* how science is supposed to work.) We've built decades of policy on weight stigma and anti-fat bias.[5]

Bodies across the weight and size spectrum can have normal blood pressure, cholesterol, blood sugar, and energy levels. Assuming that a larger body can't have normal levels is anti-fat bias, and we've been trained to believe it without question. However, when researchers suggest that a higher weight is a "risk factor" for certain diseases, they do so without evidence that a higher body weight is actually the cause. There is simply no way to state categorically that our weight is a clear indicator of our health. This is true across the body weight spectrum.

When we're concerned about our weight because the mantra "Keep it under control" has been drilled into us our entire lives, what are we to do? We diet and diet and diet and diet. Medical folks prescribe dieting over and over, even though the failure rate of weight-loss dieting is as high as 95 percent.[6] Consequently, only a few weight-loss unicorns maintained their weight loss at the

> The moral virtue we attach to health is itself very much a product of anti-fat bias (and ableism and our general relentless othering of non-ideal bodies). But if we're able to recognize **fatphobia** as a pervasive form of oppression, we should be able to stand against it regardless of whether being fat is bad for your health.
> Virginia Sole-Smith, "But What about Health?" *Burnt Toast*

three- to five-year mark, and even that weight loss didn't necessarily improve health.[7] If diets were drugs tested by the Food and Drug Administration, they would never make it to market or your doctor's prescription pad. So why do diets get recommended? You guessed it . . . weight stigma and bias.

So We Continue to Diet, Diet, and Diet

This yo-yo diet merry-go-round characterized by chronic weight loss and gain is called weight cycling. Let's break this down. When I'm working with a client on ways to move away from target weights and weight-loss plans, here's what's typically up next: "But doesn't a higher body weight increase your risk for x, y, and z?" It's pretty common to hear that people at higher weights are at greater risk for chronic diseases such as diabetes and cardiovascular disease (remember those assumptions?). What if I were to tell you that many of the issues we blame on body weight can be explained instead by weight cycling and weight stigma?

It's true. Dieting is terrible for you, no matter your body size or shape. It doesn't matter if you're young or old. Dieting is bad for your overall health.

It happens like this. The stress that weight cycling puts on the body can increase the risk of cardiovascular and renal diseases.[8] It can also increase the risk of eating disorder behaviors and lead to metabolic diseases such as diabetes. Chronic dieting also causes weight dysregulation, or weight gain beyond a person's genetic range.[9] In short, dieting may yield temporary weight loss, but it causes extra weight gain down the road. More importantly, dieting for intentional weight loss further harms overall health.

We have assumed that being at a higher weight is the single cause of most medical issues and chronic illnesses. But that isn't what the evidence shows. Although many typical weight studies do not control for chronic dieting or weight cycling, chronic dieting and weight cycling carry the blame for many of these issues. Such studies should survey each participant to collect their weight cycling and dieting history, but they don't. If they did, they might discover that the stress of dieting and weight fluctuations is also associated with poorer mental health, insulin resistance, elevated triglycerides, and abdominal fat accumulation.[10] Patients are being told over and over again to diet to "get healthy." And it is backfiring.

We're all at risk in diet culture—no matter where our weight or body size falls. No one gets out unscathed. However, dieting behaviors are most often prompted after someone has been on the receiving end of weight stigma and weight discrimination. Those facing this unjust social and medical treatment often suffer physically and psychologically.[11] People who experience repeated weight stigma, whether in their relationships, schools, workplaces, or medical offices, are also more likely to suffer from disordered eating, alcohol abuse, sleep disturbances, and a poor relationship with body movement.[12] Shame has never been an effective healthcare strategy, but it seems to be the one we use the most.

Shame has never been an effective healthcare strategy, but it seems to be the one we use the most.

We've got this health and weight stuff incredibly messed up, and we hurt people in the process. Even though we continue to promote intentional weight-loss attempts, this tactic does not improve mortality risk. In fact, weight cycling actually *increases* mortality risk.[13] What can we conclude? That chasing diet culture's weight-loss goals can lead to the risk of an earlier death. That surely doesn't sound healthy to me.

So why on God's green earth do we have to step on the scale at every single doctor's appointment? The short answer is that we don't have to consent to a weight check *at all* (more on that in part 2). The other answer has to do, once again, with weight stigma and bias in healthcare. Remember how many of us in the health and medical fields were trained in a weight-centric "care" model of health?

When we visit a medical office, we're likely to hear, "We've got to weigh you because it's a vital sign." That's a stretch. Most adults don't need to be weighed at all during medical appointments. Jennifer Gaudiani, a Denver-based physician who treats eating disorders, suggests that 90 percent of weigh-ins at medical offices are entirely unnecessary.[14] These needless weight checks often lead to lectures and shaming around body weight when a patient is actually seeking help for real medical concerns, like Jessica was.

What's a Believer to Do in a Culture That Worships Weight?

Weight is not a **behavior,** and it is largely out of our control.

Those who are believers in Jesus may wonder what they can do in response to this culture. The first step is to begin to disconnect from it. Why is it essential to question cultural ideals and beliefs? Because these norms and expectations keep us from loving ourselves, from loving our neighbors, and from implementing true health behaviors. Weight is not a behavior, and it is largely out of our control.

We must stop judging our weight and the weight of others. Can you now challenge the faulty "weight equals health" argument? Does it come from God? Or does it originate from a culture strung out on achieving ideals that were never God's ideas? We judge ourselves and others negatively based on worldly beliefs and goals. There's no love for our neighbor or love for ourselves in that judgment. Body diversity is not an accident, and it includes all colors, shapes, sizes, weights, genders, and abilities. Our weight is not a problem to fix. And it is most definitely not a significant measure of our health.

THE WORLD SAYS . . .

Your weight is your health. If you care about your health, you will "control" your weight.

THE WORD SAYS . . .

Put on the full armor of God, so that you can take your stand against the devil's schemes. For our struggle is not against flesh and blood, but against the rulers, against the authorities, against the powers of this dark world and against the spiritual forces of evil in the heavenly realms.

Ephesians 6:11–12

STEPPING AWAY FROM LIES

This may be the hardest reflection you'll be asked to undertake. It took me years to reckon with weight stigma and bias in my personal life and professional work.

- Have you judged yourself harshly in regard to your weight?

- Have you also judged others, either in your own thoughts or out loud? It's okay to admit it. We all have the seeds of weight stigma planted in our minds in this culture. The important question is, what do you want to do about it?

- You may live in a smaller body that doesn't get scrutinized in social or medical settings, and that is body privilege. We can all be harmed in this diet culture, but it's unlikely that those of us in smaller bodies have suffered like those in larger bodies have in our world. How does it feel to acknowledge this?

- If you are one of the countless victims of weight bias, does it help to know there's a name for what you've experienced? And that it's not your fault?

- Does it help to know that our culture and contemporary health policy are what have a problem, not your body?

- As you reflect on Ephesians 6:11–12, what parallels do you see between putting on the full armor of God and standing against the devil's schemes?

- How can reflecting on the teaching that "our struggle is not against flesh and blood, but against the rulers, against the authorities" help you stand against the lies about weight?

Your BMI Is a Problem

> SCIENCE: If you don't make mistakes, you're doing it wrong. If you don't correct those mistakes, you're doing it really wrong. If you can't accept that you're mistaken, you're not doing it at all.
>
> **Professor Richard Feynman, Twitter post, June 29, 2022, 2:48 a.m.**

We've heard about body mass index, or BMI, for decades now. If you thought the lies about weight were doozies, buckle up, because the BMI is even more preposterous! Our healthcare system uses it because it's viewed as a quick and dirty tool to assess health and health risks. Unfortunately, it's about as useful in determining your health as your shoe size. The BMI wasn't developed to assess individual health. It is a calculation developed by a Belgian statistician to study a *specific population of average European white men*, not individual people.

Adolphe Quetelet, also an astronomer and sociologist, was searching for a measure of the "ideal" average (white) man. That's it. Quetelet collected this information only from French and Scottish men to determine the "ideal" European man. He never intended that the equation would be used in determining health, even of those men whose information he gathered.

In her excellent book *What We Don't Talk about When We Talk about Fat*, Aubrey Gordon takes a deep dive into the racist and misogynistic roots of the BMI.[1] (I highly recommend reading her book.) The BMI was never intended to be the magic math equation that it is today, which somehow determines all individuals' health status, including races and genders not studied. Yet here we are, using it to indicate fatness and health, although it really does neither.[2]

Gordon writes, "The BMI isn't a reliable indicator of the fatness or health of people of color—not by accident, but it was never designed to be."[3] This absurd "assessment tool" causes harm to the actual health of our nation and in particular to people of color. I used to use the BMI professionally, but I've since realized how flawed it is—a tool rife with discrimination and assumptions. *The medical community didn't even use the scientific method or medical guidelines in the decision to adopt the BMI as a health indicator.* They merely followed the lead of a prominent insurance company that began using BMI to determine rate premiums.[4]

We assume that a lower BMI equals better health, while a higher BMI equals poorer health. Did you know that the BMI misclassifies nearly 75 million Americans (more than 20 percent) each year as either metabolically or cardiovascularly unhealthy or healthy?[5] That's right. The BMI is wrong a lot of the time. A study titled "Misclassification of Cardiometabolic Health When Using Body Mass Index Categories in NHANES 2005–2012" demonstrates that there are people with high BMIs in excellent cardiovascular health; at the same time, there are people with low to "normal" BMIs who have significant metabolic dysregulation and disease. These same researchers suggest that focusing on BMI and weight to improve health is ineffective and harmful.[6] When we use BMI as a proxy for health, we all suffer. *Please, dear Lord, make it go away.*

When we use **BMI** as a proxy for health, we all suffer.

The Harm of Using the BMI to Assess Health

I introduced you to Teri in the introduction. I was fortunate to meet her in the early years of her eating disorder treatment and recovery process. When Teri and I began working together, she thought she simply didn't know how to diet "the right way." What she didn't realize, because she had never been assessed, was that her chronic restriction and dieting was an eating disorder.

Teri came to see me every week at first. Each time, I'd learn more and more about her life, her struggles, her kids, and her support network. She had been the victim of medical weight stigma so many times in her life. Weight loss was often on her mind, but she now knew that by pursuing it, she had ended up with an eating disorder. Knowing that, however, didn't make it easier to stop thinking about weight loss, especially since her doctor encouraged her at every single appointment to lose weight.

After Teri and I had worked together for about six months, she began to focus less on losing weight and more on nourishing her body, regardless of how her body weight may respond. She stabilized her eating pattern by eating regular meals and snacks, getting support from her family, and reducing her stress at work, so we thought it would be a good time to space her appointments out to every couple of weeks.

The next time I saw her, she was distraught. She had been horribly ill with a prolonged stomach bug, one so severe that she twice needed IV fluids in the emergency room. She had only been able to start eating normally again a few days before she came back to see me. Teri had a follow-up appointment with her physician just before her session in my office.

EATING DISORDERS STATISTICS

Eating disorders do not have a look, gender, race, or body weight. Any person can suffer from an eating disorder. The Association of Anorexia Nervosa and Associated Disorders shares these statistics:

- *Less than 6 percent* of those diagnosed with an eating disorder are "underweight."
- Eating disorders affect almost 10 percent of the world's population.
- Black, Indigenous, and People of Color are *half as likely* to be diagnosed with or receive treatment for an eating disorder.
- Women with physical disabilities are more likely to develop an eating disorder in their lifetime.[7]

Teri sat down and pulled the box of tissues closer, and she wept. When she was ready to talk, she told me about the experience at her doctor's office earlier that morning. Like so many health professionals, her physician didn't think she had an eating disorder because of her body size. Therefore, the doctor congratulated her on her weight loss instead of being concerned about her eating disorder, recent stomach bug, and electrolyte irregularities.

When Teri reminded the doctor that her weight loss was due to a violent and long-lasting stomach bug, her doctor remained unconcerned. She continued with her summary, telling me that as she was pulling herself together to leave the office, the doctor leaned out of the exam room door and said, "Hey, don't be sad. Your BMI is lower; that's great news!"

Teri was utterly stunned. It wasn't just that the doctor was out of line with the unsolicited comment and complete disregard of her recent illness; it was that Teri knew she was a Jesus follower by the cross that hung around her neck. Teri said she felt judged and hurt. This wasn't just an attack on her weight; she perceived it as an attack on her worth. She cried the entire ten-mile trip to my office.

Eric had a similar experience. He was thirteen the first time he came to my office. His dad sat next to him at our first visit and told me about how his son's eating disorder started. The boy's coach—a family friend and fellow churchgoer—had done weight checks at the team practice and told the boy his BMI was too high. This coach also gave him advice on how to bring it down by engaging in overexercise and undereating.

For most kids, coaches have a huge amount of influence, much like that of a parent, aunt, uncle, or caregiver. It is rarely appropriate for a coach to weigh a child or give nutrition advice beyond "It's important for you to show up at practice fed and hydrated." This advice and nonsense BMI talk sent Eric into a two-year battle to salvage his physical and mental health. Eric suffered because of faulty "health tools" and a coach who gave poor, inappropriate advice.

Both Teri and Eric were wounded in what they thought

It is rarely appropriate for a coach to weigh a child or give **nutrition advice** beyond "It's important for you to show up at practice fed and hydrated."

were safe places by those whom they thought were safe people. Most likely, Teri's doctor and Eric's coach *thought* they were helping. (I know because I've been that not-so-safe person.) Sometimes we don't know what we don't know.

Even When We Do Know, We Must Do Better

The BMI is garbage for adults, but it is a blazing dumpster fire for children. When a person is constantly growing and developing, using the BMI is like trying to hit a moving target. Because childhood is such a volatile time of growth, with increases in all bodily tissues, the BMI misclassifies children as well.[8] And even though a randomized clinical trial (the very best kind of study) concluded that BMI report cards in schools aren't helpful and even promote body dissatisfaction, many schools still use this practice.[9]

The BMI is a flawed math equation and a relic of racist oppression. There are no scientific indications that it is a useful medical tool to use on individuals. When providers understand this fact, that is knowledge; when we know the truth and continue to use the BMI, that is a weapon.

As I write this chapter, our government funding agencies are pouring billions of taxpayer dollars into ob*sity research, even though decades of evidence suggest the harm and futility of weight-loss dieting.[10] Our current medical and health system seems fully invested in continuing to use the BMI as a health assessment tool because it is inextricably tied to diagnosing people with ob*sity. Remember, diet culture is in the so-called "safe" places. There's a lot of money to be made if we continue to tell people that shrinking is the only way to health.

A diagnosis of ob*sity (based on the BMI) may mean more billable insurance codes and drug options, but it's an unlikely path to health or well-being. Body size hasn't always been labeled a disease, but the choice to make it a disease surely has been a lucrative one.

Remember when I told you this gets even crazier? Here we go. The American Obesity Society declared "excess" body fat, or ob*sity, a disease in 2008.[11] In 2012, the American Medical Association (AMA), the most prestigious and influential medical association in our country, charged its science and public health council to evaluate the evidence. Their job was to determine if ob*sity was a disease. *The council did not find sufficient evidence to support calling "excess" body fat a disease.*

> **Body size hasn't always been labeled a disease, but the choice to make it a disease surely has been a lucrative one.**

At the time, the AMA assumed that calling ob*sity a disease would positively impact health policy, insurance reimbursement, and industry funding. The association also thought it would open the door for expanded research into what causes people to have larger bodies and to find ways to prevent them. (I'm fuming, by the way, because body diversity comes from God.) Instead of accepting the report that concluded there is insufficient evidence to deem body weight a disease, the AMA moved forward with a vote. And in June 2013, nonconforming body size, or "ob*sity," became a diagnosis.[12]

We've built an entire war on bodies *based on a vote*—a vote on making body size a disease based not on evidence but on the bias rampant in diet culture. Dr. Maggie Landes, a Texas-based physician who educates other professionals about the harm of weight stigma in the practice of medicine, says it best: "If that's not the most flagrant example of weight stigma derailing the entire practice of medicine, I'm not sure what is! The AMA asked for the evidence, and they flatly rejected it in favor of upholding what is proven to be a discriminatory and unethical model of clinical practice."[13]

This vote made it medically acceptable to add stigmatizing labels to humans who live in larger bodies. And it has not improved our nation's health—just the opposite. As my colleague Jennifer Gaudiani, MD, said in a *Food Psych* podcast conversation with Christy Harrison, "Physicians are constantly talking about the so-called 'obesity epidemic' . . . and I'm pretty sure we're the ones who caused it."[14] Weight stigma and bias only cause harm. It is real trauma. I pray we can start to mend together.

THE WORLD SAYS . . .

If you live in a body larger than our cultural ideal, it is wrong and needs to be changed.

THE WORD SAYS . . .

See to it that no one takes you captive through hollow and deceptive philosophy, which depends on human tradition and the elemental spiritual forces of this world rather than on Christ.

Colossians 2:8

STEPPING AWAY FROM LIES

Our world and human traditions can be incredibly challenging, especially if you feel like you don't fit in.

- How does it make you feel to know we're waging a war on divinely created bodies?

- Did learning about the history of the BMI's development help you see its futility and harm?

- It's possible you've experienced harm like both Teri and Eric did. If you feel safe to think back about this, can you claim that your body is not wrong? Can you attribute this experience to deceptive philosophy and harmful human traditions?

- If you've been like the doctor or the coach in these cases and caused harm because of what you learned in diet culture, can you allow yourself the grace to move forward with change? Remember, I've done this too.

- If you're a church leader or Bible study leader and you've used weight or BMI in your lessons to push change in your congregation or group members, can you see the secular influence and potential to cause harm?

- Be sure to offer yourself grace moving forward. If we are to receive this grace, we can no longer let these deceptive philosophies creep in. Spend some time thinking about Colossians 2:8.

Diet Culture Lie #8

Health Lessons Teach Health

When I talk to eating disorder professionals, I ask: How many of you have clients whose eating disorder was triggered or worsened by a school "nutrition" lesson? Every. Hand. Goes. Up.

Every. Time.

Katja Rowell, MD, responsive feeding specialist and author

Ben still remembers when his health class teacher made him and his classmates count their calories for a grade. He also remembers when the teacher suggested that the students cut calories and fat in their diets so they could be "healthier." This was the tipping point, Ben said. Slowly, he began counting more calories and eating less food. His teacher, family, and church friends congratulated him on his diet changes. And then he collapsed. After Ben's hospitalization for malnutrition and an irregular heart rhythm, I started working with him to help him unlearn what he had learned in health class.

Ben is one of so many who have suffered at the hands of our diet culture–infested education system. There are far too many stories to tell here. The horrifying experiences of health class harm could fill volumes of books. You may have suffered this way as well—in a health class, a Bible study lesson on "wellness," or a well-meaning conversation in a fitness session. You may have witnessed something like this recently. I'm guessing you're starting to see diet culture in the "safe" places a lot more.

When I think about the most common places these messages show up and plant seeds of doubt, I reflect on health lessons in schools. Like so many of us, teachers grew up in a culture rife with teachings of self-doubt and body distrust. They likely learned in their studies that less food is healthy (it's not) and bigger bodies are wrong (they're not). Like the rest of us, they may have even picked up traditions in their own home or church around food and body restriction and righteousness. Teachers also suffer from the lies of diet culture and unknowingly pass them along to their students. Now we have trickle-down harm.

Both of my parents were teachers who worked tirelessly for their students. Please understand that I'm not trying to pick on teachers. Teachers are a crucial part of our lives who shouldn't be forced to share harmful misinformation. They have a tremendous opportunity to see diet culture and keep it out of their classrooms—and we can support them in doing so.

It Starts Sooner Than We Think

My daughter was two years old when she began attending a parents' day out program at a local church. It was such a sweet program. The kids learned as much as toddlers can learn about Jesus. They learned about kindness and sharing. And they learned which foods came with a warning—"You can have ice cream and Easter candy, but *not too much*."

Not long after viewing the "good food, bad food" villains on the kids television channel, I realized we would have to talk about diet culture very early in our home. We settled on the phrase "health propaganda" to call out the lies of diet culture. According to Merriam-Webster's online dictionary, *propaganda* is defined as "the spreading of ideas, information, or rumor for the purpose of helping or injuring an institution, a cause, or a person." The cause, in this case, is diet culture, which helps the diet industry continue to profit through its oppression of bodies. We must call out health propaganda whenever and wherever we see it.

If you have a child in a school program, you may have been given requirements or restrictions on sending food to school—requirements that assume a family has the money to buy those foods, values consumption of certain foods, and has a child who will happily accept the foods. Even though most schools have very little, if any, idea about a family's financial abilities or cultural values regarding food, food lists are often sent home with specific guidelines. A school may limit the calories of a snack brought from home. They may advise staying under x grams of sugar or restrict certain snack foods. Some programs may go so far as to allow only fruits and vegetables as snacks.

In these cases, diet culture sets a perilous boundary that doesn't foster a child's body autonomy or support independence around the foods a family accepts and can afford. This type of diet culture training is happening before our children are even able to go to the bathroom on their own. These lessons repeatedly affirm to children that they must not trust their own instincts around food or their bodies. They become seeds of doubt planted in what is supposed to be a "safe" place. And many more seeds are being scattered.

When a child sits independently at a lunch table, lunch box policing may start. Perhaps it's a well-meaning parent volunteer, a school lunch monitor, a principal, or even another child. This policing may begin as another list or food rule-ish suggestions. Your child may hear phrases like, "Eat your growing foods first," "You can have that after you eat your fruit," or "Only one cookie." None of these well-meaning comments are built on evidence. They've been manufactured in diet culture and have become an elementary school tradition. These statements don't help the health of our children; rather, they make them question their bodies and the food available to them.

You may be thinking these comments are helpful for guiding children toward more nutritious options. And that thought makes sense, because all parents want their children to have a variety of foods that provide great nutrition. It's one thing for teachers to say no soda in the classroom to avoid spills that might attract bugs, or no birthday foods because of food allergies, but it's a whole other can of food-shaming worms to say no to "junk food"—a term of opinion—in the classroom. I've been in the classroom where the only food option for a child to bring for lunch was a small bag of chips. Another child with feeding difficulties brings chips for a snack because it's one of just a few accepted foods. The chips are not "junk"; they are the food that allows the child to be fed.

The first goal of nutrition is to be fed—adequately

> **The first goal of nutrition is to be fed—adequately and consistently.**

and consistently. Now, I'm not saying that children can't benefit from a variety of foods. I'd love to see all schools have access to a wide variety of foods that are offered to children without shame or pressure. But that isn't what children are getting, and that's not always how food is offered.

Children accept what feels safe, and when broccoli or carrots taste okay one time and slimy the next, the inconsistency can be scary. It's no wonder children often prefer packaged and familiar foods; they're never a surprise to them. When we speak negatively about foods our kids may prefer, we make them question what has made them feel safe, fed, and confident.

After a child has heard the "eat this food first" message for a few years, we don't have to call other foods bad or lesser; the message has already been implied and absorbed. So when the reading lessons include the dichotomizing of foods into healthy and unhealthy categories, there is minimal questioning—until now, because now you can spot the lies of diet culture and help call out health propaganda. When the homework suggests the shopper is healthy because their grocery cart contains fruit, I hope you'll stop and think about this assignment. Is this shopper healthy because of what is in their cart? Or are they capable of affording those groceries? What's in their cart gives no other information, especially information that can provide insight into their health status. This is a lesson about privilege, not health.

Dichotomizing Happens All the Time in School Lessons

Good versus bad food examples show up in nearly every subject because this philosophy is written into core curriculums. Teachers are urged to instruct their students about healthy choices in diet culture terms and are given no alternatives. They often have to

pull lessons from canned or free programs to meet the requirements. And in so doing, they may unknowingly perpetuate a
"good food, bad food" approach. Children who learn dichoto-
mized food messages may ultimately conclude they are bad for
desiring foods that don't fit into the good food category. I have
never seen this translate to a healthy
relationship with their food or body
down the road. In fact, I've seen in
my practice that most people who
struggle with food received damaging messages about food, eating, and
bodies in their childhood—messages
that can be extremely difficult to overcome as an adult.

> Children who learn
> dichotomized food
> messages may
> ultimately conclude
> they are **bad** for
> desiring foods
> that don't fit into
> the **good** food
> category.

When teachers aren't provided with
better alternatives, they use whatever they
can find to meet the standards. In recent years,
the resources include documentaries about food,
bodies, and health. Next to calorie-counting assignments, documentaries have caused the most harm to
my school-aged clients. Documentaries are profoundly compel-
ling. They cleverly cite and misconstrue research studies just
enough to make us question what we're doing with our food and
bodies. But know this: documentaries are not science; they're
entertainment, designed to sway people's opinion. These types
of films about "health and nutrition" have no place in schools.
I even strongly caution my adult clients and friends against
watching them. These documentaries all too often are examples
of health propaganda.

As our children are exposed to these lessons, they're also
learning about dichotomizing bodies. In books, bad or unpopular
characters may appear in larger bodies, while the hero is depicted

as trim and muscular. Some lessons may include language imply-ing that bigger bodies are less "healthy" than smaller ones or that makes assumptions about the eating habits of those in smaller or larger bodies. Illustrations tend to show only certain types of "healthy" bodies—those that are thin, White, and able-bodied. We don't have to explicitly teach kids to internalize the ideal of diet culture for them to carry that bias into the future. This false belief will cause harm to themselves and to others.

As our children enter middle school, which is already a challenging time due to pubertal changes, assignments change from reading about "hypothetical students" in class to evaluat-ing our children's own bodies, such as what happened with Ben. *How much do you weigh? How many calories do you eat? Let's evaluate whether it's too many calories according to our usual dieting [read "starvation"] standards. How long would it take to lose x number of pounds with this math? Would it be healthy if you gained weight? Or if you lost weight?*

This is an explosive season of growth and development—a season when weight gain and growth should be normalized, not demonized.

In this season, assignments often include stepping on the scale in the classroom as part of a lesson or mis-guided state health initiatives. In no way are these assignments about health. In a culture that weaponizes weight, there is no school weight check that is appro-priate or that will bring benefit rather than cause harm. The chosen philosophy centers around all the flawed values and assumptions we uphold in diet culture. As a parent, teacher,

> In a culture that **weaponizes** weight, there is no school weight check that is appropriate or that will bring benefit rather than cause harm.

guardian, or friend, you can draw a line in the sand. You can let children know before they're even exposed to diet culture and dichotomizing food messages that they can opt out. They can say no and deny consent.

You Will Learn Untruths

I say, "You will learn untruths," a lot in my home. My daughter tells me about something she read at school or heard another adult or child say in passing. Whenever I ask her what untruths she has heard lately, she's never short on examples. As we have family conversations about diet culture, we also have to realize that we can't protect our loved ones from all the ways it will show up in their lives. Speaking truth to the untruths is the only way to build resilience in our lives and in our culture. We must

UNTRUTH AND TRUTH CONVERSATIONS

Here are a few examples of untruth and truth conversations I've had with my daughter and with clients who identify as Jesus followers—conversations about body diversity and diet culture that take place regularly these days. Remember that it's okay if this topic is new to you. Take your time. You don't have to get every conversation right. I often don't. But we do have to try.

Messages of Untruth	Conversations around Truth
"My teacher said I only need to eat fruit for a snack."	"That is an untruth. Thank you for sharing this with me. What do you think about that statement? Does our family believe there is only one way to eat? Do you think all families can offer only fruit as a snack? Do you like other foods for snacks? The truth is that there is no rule about snacks."

"We talked about the word *healthy* at Sunday school today. Our teachers said that means not eating too much and keeping a healthy weight."	"Thank you for sharing this with me. What you were told sounds untrue. Do you think God is worried about the food on your plate (besides that you're getting enough, of course)? Do you think God made all bodies—big, small, and colorful—on purpose? Do you think God cares more about a number on a scale than about your heart? Your Sunday school teacher lives in diet culture too. I'm happy to chat with them about this if you'd like me to."
"Our health teacher said we need to write down our food intake and weigh ourselves to stay healthy."	"Does that sound like truth to you? Do you believe a great God would make our bodies so hard to manage? I'm curious if you think these ideas are actually healthy. Would you like to tell your teacher you're not going to participate, or would you like me to contact them? This untruth will harm you and your friends as well."

have hard conversations with this generation to have any hope that the next generation will be different.

When the lies of diet culture invade medical offices and schools, they receive even more power. Our culture holds these prescriptions, messages, and lessons in high esteem, sometimes elevating them above the words of God and often craftily wrapping them in Scripture verses. We must be careful not to confuse the untruths of the world with the truth that sets us free. The truth is this: our weight and health are not prerequisites for receiving the love of God. Our weight and health have nothing to do with our worthiness in the kingdom of God. The same goes for our kids.

THE WORLD SAYS . . .

Health is something you can learn
about, micromanage, and achieve
if you believe our lessons.

THE WORD SAYS . . .

This is what the LORD Almighty says:
"Do not listen to what the prophets are
prophesying to you;
they fill you with false hopes.
They speak visions from their own minds,
not from the mouth of the LORD."

Jeremiah 23:16

STEPPING AWAY FROM LIES

- Do you remember "health" lessons such as the ones described in this chapter?

- Do you hear about your kids' health teachings from them?

- You may have taught some of these lessons yourself. I'm curious how this chapter may have stirred you. Please know you're not alone in this. No one is out to shame you. Don't forget that my early professional experience included peddling and teaching diet culture.

- Knowing now that health isn't just a lesson in diet culture or something we can work really hard to achieve, what will you do with this information?

- As you reflect on Jeremiah 23:16, do you see parallels of false hopes and false prophets in our society today?

Your Weight Secures Your Righteousness

> Wherever there is food, there is diet culture. And there is a lot of food in church.
>
> **Dr. Erin Bowers, associate pastor, First Presbyterian Church, High Point, North Carolina**

For years I've wrestled with the way diet culture shows up to attack believers. Because church members are immersed in this culture, along with everyone else, we can be assured it *will* show up. Believers will diet. Influential Christian leaders will continue to sell nutrition plans, sugar detoxes, and straight-up diets wrapped in Bible verses. In fact, one of the most common places where people sell multilevel marketing (MLM) diet plans, complete with shakes and snack bars, is church. The church should be the safest of all the "safe" places, but diet culture sits very comfortably in its pews.

Haven't most of us been on a diet at some point in our

lives? Of course we've dieted! We've
been sold lies about dieting, food,
and bodies our entire lives. We're
programmed to think we *have* to be
dieters in this culture. I don't have
a problem with people thinking they
need to diet; I do have a problem with
the church suggesting that it's a path to
righteousness. I have a problem with the
church deceptively making weight, which is
an issue of this world, an issue of the Word.
But we can't see the deception because it's
wrapped up with "health" and false virtue.

> The church should
> be the **safest** of
> all the "safe" places,
> but diet culture sits
> very comfortably
> in its pews.

The enemy loves diet culture within the community of believers. As long as the church permits
diet culture to advance unchecked, it will allow weight bias and
racism to remain within its walls. A congregation that worships
diet culture's thin ideal will be incapable of loving neighbors
who don't look the part. When we're chasing the weight of this
world, we will fail to love our bodies and souls and those of
others as well. There is no way to offer our neighbors what we
don't have for ourselves. Our weight has nothing to do with our
righteousness; our neighbor's body has nothing to do with their
righteousness either.

We Must Evict This Weight and Worthiness Way of Thinking

How have we not seen the deception? I believe it's because of
the pedestal on which we've placed our medical system—an
infallible, godlike pedestal. As you reflect on the last couple
of chapters, I hope you can see how the health and medical

fields are most definitely not infallible because, after all, we're all human. Please don't read this and think I believe health providers are ignorant, awful people, because I don't—I'm a health provider myself. But medical providers have an ethical obligation to do no harm. Furthermore, if you're a Christian medical provider, I believe you have an overarching responsibility to *love your neighbor* (your patient) and *do no harm*. Prescribing more of the same diet culture interventions is not loving our neighbor or preventing harm.

> **Prescribing more of the same diet culture interventions is not loving our neighbor or preventing harm.**

Those in medical professions, just as those in positions of influence in churches and schools, have been brought up in diet culture. There is no way we can be swayed away unless we've been stirred by those who fought the battles before us or we've come to realize we harmed someone and have resolved to change our approach. I got lucky to have the opportunity to unlearn. I also harmed.

Along the way, I learned the hierarchy within the health and medical professions. Yes, doctors go to school for what seems like a gazillion years, and I have enormous appreciation for them and their skills. And our culture often treats their words as gospel truth. In elevating doctors in such a way, we've put extraordinary pressure on them to be our infallible saviors.

This cultural occupational hierarchy has opened the door for Christian leaders to elevate doctors on par with spiritual advisers—and sometimes even higher. A pastor may say we only need a doctor and a preacher to guide our major decisions. Your church may promote books and programs written by pastors and doctors to encourage dieting or adopting a certain lifestyle as a way to godliness, worthiness, and righteousness. Listen, I get it—I want everyone to have good information. I have the utmost respect for the physicians and pastors in my circles, but no one has all the information. And I can tell you, not one of the collaborative programs I've seen wasn't strongly influenced by diet culture.

I recently caught wind of a new spiritual "health" program that targets children. It is supported by a ministry leader and a well-known doctor on social media. The program's marketing suggests that its goal is to teach children that it's wrong to desire foods like cookies. A program like this is inappropriate for kids, as are most nutrition-based programs; it ties hunger and the desire to eat pleasurable foods to their goodness and obedience to God. But this is not a health program; it is a recipe for an eating disorder wrapped up in "righteousness," not to mention lifelong worries about their worthiness and whether God loves them! I know; I've been on the "aftermath treatment" side of this type of program for decades.

This approach seems similar to sermons I've heard on "dying to the flesh" from Bible passages such as Romans 8:13–14. That makes sense when we're trying to avoid drinking too much. The body doesn't need alcohol to live. But when a church leader gives advice about what we can and cannot eat, the potential is there for the flesh to, quite literally, die. We were designed to need food, and not all believers have access to the same foods. Flesh must be fed. Sadly, we've learned in this culture that flesh that doesn't look the part must be altered.

> We were designed to **need food,** and not all believers have access to the same foods.

Some leaders get right to the point and suggest that weight loss invariably makes us righteous, no matter how we get there. Any program will work if we just pray for more willpower. We can pray over our scale a little harder this time. Sometimes leaders share a fad diet that worked (temporarily) for them and start promoting it to their following. They may throw in a few prayers and notable Bible verses for good Christian measure. This happens all the time—the "it worked for me so I'm sure you can do it too" diet. This leader may have privileges and resources their followers don't have, like an unlimited grocery budget and the kind of time needed to participate in these programs. And they certainly have differences in genetics. We are not all the same.

I see this scenario play out all too often in my circles. What will happen to the leader's followers who fail to lose weight or maintain their weight loss by any means necessary? What will happen to the followers who trusted their leader to draw them closer to Christ in the "thirty-day diet for holiness" challenge? They end up staying in the diet culture shame cycle. They end up enduring the diet aftermath. You see, now they haven't just failed the leader who wrapped a diet in a Bible verse and made it seem so doable (just have faith); they've also failed God. Oh, how damaging and wrong!

Then in sneaky diet culture fashion, we move away from the programs that call themselves diets. Remember, it's a lifestyle or healthy eating plan now, and this "not a diet diet" is a lifestyle for Jesus. Oh, and—wink, wink—you might lose weight. This plan is wrapped in a different verse but comes with a list of foods you can and can't eat—and these aren't just run-of-the-mill foods either. To be obedient in these plans, you have to sacrifice even more resources than you may be comfortable with. So not only is it another diet; it's only for those who can afford the ministry's medically approved list of foods. Righteousness is only for those who can pay for it in this plan. If it's not an option for everyone, I can't believe God requires it for anyone.

We've also seen the emergence of detoxes in Christian spaces. Sometimes detoxes are dressed up like Lenten practices; other times they're part of just a straight-up diet du jour avoidance of a food or ingredient. The church has become so wrapped up in diet culture that we think an all-powerful God who made every single thing, including us, can't handle little ingredients like sugar.

God created plants. Sugar cane is a plant. Glucose, a simple form of sugar, is the preferred fuel source for our brains.[1] God gave humans the power to turn all things into food. God made our bodies. We are sacred. But now diet culture dictates the way we care for ourselves and judge others. And so we go on another diet, lifestyle plan, detox, or fast, believing it may bring us closer to something sacred, while in reality it is all too often at the service of diet culture.

You Can Be Set Free

Perhaps you're on a diet or following a health plan right now. You decided the information you were given in the "safe" places could be trusted. Maybe the information came from your pastor or your parents, or maybe it came from the Christian teacher you follow on social media. Those teachers have given us so much excellent information and may have even helped us draw closer to God. But I'm afraid they've been led astray when it comes to bodies, health, and food, just like the rest of us have. Though they meant well, they led us down a misguided path.

But I have good news. We can be set free when we realize that our bodies have nothing to do with our righteousness. The number on a bathroom scale will not determine worth or virtue, but it will most definitely distract us from living for the glory of God. How can we be the hands and feet of Christ when all we can think about is what we can't eat and how our calorie intake may change the reading on that metal device on the bathroom floor?

Focus on the scale and weight equates to idol worship. I pray that our ministry leaders and Christian influencers will recognize this. Though pastors and church leaders generally have a great deal of knowledge and a deep love for the Lord, they aren't trained health professionals (unless they are, of course)—and even then, we've already outlined the problems with education in the health professions. As you've gathered from previous chapters, most of us in healthcare aren't being taught to see the big picture.

We engage in idol worship when we obsess over the bathroom scale and become focused on our weight.

Between office visits, my clients and I will sometimes send emails back and forth to ask and answer quick questions or share concerns—things like, "Leslie, I'm just staring at my food and I don't know what to do." I feel the hurt in their words. On too many occasions, clients have emailed to tell me about a diet their pastor mentioned or a small group Bible study where the goal for the year was to start a new diet plan. Other times, the voices of their past haunt the present care of their bodies. They may have heard that eating certain foods, having a certain body type, or being a certain weight made them poor stewards of their bodies. At the same time they're working with me to free themselves from the diet- and weight-obsessed world, they're continually being confronted with the effects of diet culture teaching in a place where our best efforts at unconditional love should be experienced.

Our bodies are a gift from God. Taking care of these divine gifts allows us to do the work of Jesus in this world. But it doesn't look the same for everyone. And it doesn't look like our culture's typical "health" practices. In part 2, we'll talk a lot more about what health does and doesn't look like. Until then, think about this: as long as we equate weight with health and righteousness, we'll impede the work that could be done in the name of Jesus, and we'll continue to harm each other.

THE WORLD SAYS . . .

A number on the scale secures your righteousness.

THE WORD SAYS . . .

Do not turn to idols or make metal gods
for yourselves. I am the LORD your God.

Leviticus 19:4

STEPPING AWAY FROM LIES

The sacred and the secular have become deeply intertwined. It's true, of course, that Christians cannot withdraw from the world; Jesus came to a broken world to save us from our sin. The sacred and the secular will invariably interact, which at times makes perfect sense—for example, when we love our neighbor, whether or not they are believers. Other times, we wrap up earthly beliefs and make them seem sacred—for example, when the spheres of medicine and ministry are coupled (dangerously so) in the arena of diet culture.

- What surprised you in this chapter?

- Did any of the descriptions of diet programs, "lifestyle" plans, detoxes, and the like stand out to you?

- Have you participated in any of these programs, or do you know of others who have? What kind of feelings do you have about that?

- What challenges might you face if you chose to evict the number on the scale from your view of righteousness or worthiness?

- Read Leviticus 19:4. Would you consider the scale an idol in your life?

- If you knew that a number on a scale really doesn't have anything to do with being a good steward of your body, would that change your mind about your approach to health?

- Would you be willing to get rid of the scales in your home? Journal a bit deeper on that answer.

We're All Just Gluttons in the Temple

We will not find freedom and wholeness this side of heaven if our churches and communities teach women, overtly or subtly, to be disdainful of and/or fearful of their own bodies.

Jess Connolly, *Breaking Free from Body Shame*

You may feel that it doesn't matter what you've chosen to do when it comes to food—that ultimately you're going to fail. Jane felt that way. She told me she had accomplished a lot in her life. A great career, loving children, and good friendships. Her life was full. She made an appointment with me because she felt gluttony was the one thing in life she couldn't overcome.

Jane shared her history of growing up in a family with food security, but certain foods, such as sweets, potato chips, and anything full-fat, were not allowed in her home. Later in life, her partner shamed her when she ate certain foods or took seconds.

In her family's home and church, she learned that her body size was a sign of her disobedience. She couldn't help but link her food and body struggles to what she perceived to be spiritual failure. Jane's experiences growing up and in her early relationships heightened her belief that curing her gluttony would help her move forward with her life.

Early one morning, Jane came to her appointment in good spirits and shared that she had been feeding herself regularly and adequately. She realized that she felt like she had great energy and was having fewer episodes of uncontrollable eating at night (her "gluttony"). As we dug into what she'd been experiencing during years of trying to control her eating, I realized that Jane wasn't suffering from gluttony; rather, she was underfed. All those nights of eating what felt like too much was her very wise body urging her to get more food because it needed the fuel, not because Jane was greedy. She was experiencing the normal desires of a hungry body, not the forces of gluttony. Honoring that hunger is how she survived.

Diet culture leads us to believe that feeling out of control with food is related to our willpower, righteousness, or capabilities. That is a lie. Can you imagine growing up without diet culture, without ever having heard that your body or food was tied to your worthiness? If these seeds had not been planted, it's likely you wouldn't be fearing body change or whether you'll have enough of this or that food. You would have trusted your divine design from the get-go.

Diet culture has invaded the sacred space where our inner wisdom resides. If you had never known guilt around eating decisions, food selection, or self-care, would you have ever labeled yourself or someone else a glutton? Jane fed her body in amounts that sometimes felt frantic and uncomfortable because she had been restricting a body that needed more nourishment than a dieting culture allowed. Her body was wise, but diet culture wouldn't let her believe it.

What Is a Glutton?

I have never met a glutton in more than two decades in nutrition therapy practice. Never. Not even one. But I've met countless people who thought they were because of our culture's teaching about food, bodies, and desire. The diet cycle keeps us thinking that the pendulum from "purity" to "screw it" makes us gluttons. Nothing could be further from the truth. Pleasure and food are gifts of God. The desire for nourishment is from God. The fear that you're a glutton, which entangles you in the dieting ways of this world, is not from God.

Diet culture has invaded the **sacred space** *where our inner wisdom resides.*

If we're not gluttons simply because we desire food, then what is a glutton? Well, the simplest definition I can find suggests that a glutton is someone who enjoys excess or is overindulgent. In my studies of this word, the most common synonym is *greedy*. It makes sense that we think gluttony only has to do with food and eating because "eating in excess" is the most common example. Note that it is the example, *not the definition*. Gluttony is the greedy hoarding of things that results in taking from others.

Think back to early in the COVID pandemic when toilet paper was a hot commodity. Some people bought a bunch of packs and stored them in their garages for themselves—and in some cases even to sell at exorbitant prices. This is an example of gluttonous behavior. In the Bible, the word *gluttony* is used to refer to excess. This word is often associated with feasting and drinking wine. Imagine a party where the hosts hoard the grains, meats, fruits, vegetables, oils, and wines while the hungry and needy sit just outside the door. To me, that's another example of gluttony. Gluttony is a heart problem, not a "what you eat" or "how you eat" problem.

Church leaders must stop packaging gluttony in sermons about our food and bodies—messages that perpetuate diet culture beliefs in the church and tend to cause harm to the body. I interviewed a wise theologian and diet culture–informed pastor who told me that gluttony essentially involves taking more than our share or hoarding in a way that doesn't allow access to others. Eating in a way that makes us feel too full when having food availability after being restricted (typical undereating and dieting) or not having access to enough food (food insecurity) is not gluttonous behavior; it is survival.

Eating in a way that causes us to feel too full at our Thanksgiving feasts shouldn't be described as gluttonous. In fact, Jesus' first miracle took place at a wedding feast (John 2). Feasting with family and friends allows us to celebrate and to express gratitude for God's good gifts. However, in doing so, sometimes we feel too full, which can lead to feeling guilty. I wonder if the guilt we feel regarding that full feeling at large meals or celebrations comes from the restrictions imposed by diet culture—*I shouldn't eat this. I'll take just one spoonful, just one little bite.* Being fed—consistently and adequately—is required to support our divine design and to celebrate it.

We can't talk about the word *gluttony* without addressing the scoop of judgment that weight bias via diet culture has heaped on believers. When we feel these judgments creep in, we can challenge our thoughts and hearts. Our culture taught weight bias to us at a young age, maybe even at Sunday school. We may not think we judge others, but we do. Making assumptions about the size of someone's body tells us nothing about their eating habits, overall health, or love for God. It only shows us the posture of our own hearts. We must stop attaching the word *gluttony* to bodies, for it is a judgment that is not ours to give.

> Making assumptions about the size of someone's body tells us nothing about their eating habits, overall health, or love for God. It only shows us the posture of our own **hearts.**

Where Does Reassessing Gluttony Leave Our Temples?

If there is one verse that has been taken out of context to endorse diet culture in the church, it is 1 Corinthians 6:19: "Do you not know that your bodies are temples of the Holy Spirit, who is in you, whom you have received from God? You are not your own."

This verse isn't referring to the eating of cookies, meats, or grains—or any food, for that matter. If we read 1 Corinthians 6 in its context and refer to reputable commentaries, we'll *never* find any indication that Paul meant we should be concerned about weight or diet when he wrote, "Your bodies are temples of the Holy Spirit."[1] Pastor and theologian Erin Kesterton Bowers says, "Some pastors and theologians may have interpreted this passage to refer to food, body weight, and the like—but when that happens, it seems to me what is going on is that they are looking at this verse through the lens of diet culture rather than in its context. And this is just another way that when we approach Scripture, we have to challenge what we've learned and how it has been culturally conditioned."[2]

Our bodies are temples, not because of what we do for them, but because they *already* hold the divine. We must feed them to live with purpose. We must feed them adequately and consistently if we can. What we provide them matters, but not to the extent that we've been taught (remember the social determinants of health?). Have we forgotten that nothing can separate us from God's love? We have allowed our view of the Bible to be distorted by the lens of diet culture. Messages around food and our bodies, enfolded skillfully in verses from the Bible, have been used in nefarious ways. It's time to clean our lenses.

Even though the "our bodies are temples" verse is not about food selection or consumption, some people use it to suggest that the particular way we eat food is a reflection of morality. We were born with a need for nourishment. Feeding our bodies is in no way a moral or immoral act. It is, however, a unique experience for each of us, meaning it does not look the same for everyone. Would we be taking care of our individual divine design if it did?

Imagine that you follow a churchy social media health guru who suggests you should only put certain foods in your "temple" because your body "is not your own." This guru advises fueling your temple with such foods as organic berries, wild-caught fish, ancient grains, green smoothies, and acai bowls (feel free to eat these foods if you want, but just know it doesn't make you a holier person). A costly buy-in to the churchy health guru program will give you access to their exclusive grocery list. Following their way will ensure that your temple stays in tip-top shape for God.

You buy all the things. You may even feel a little more righteous for doing so. After all, it's about keeping your temple in check. But what if you don't even know about this plan? What if you can't buy all the things? What if you aren't on social media because you feel like it sucks your soul dry and you want to protect it? What if you don't have a smartphone? What if you don't have the money to feed yourself or your family adequately? What if you don't have a table to sit at to eat? Is your temple less worthy? No, it's most assuredly not, because 1 Corinthians 6:19 has nothing to do with feeding ourselves.

To be sure, many people have the best of intentions, but we are missing the point of grace. Every bit of nonsense we've seen about this verse and its supposed application to food is a diet culture lie. The perpetuation of this lie creates a further divide between believers who have and believers who have not. We have the love of a great God in common, but that's the only assumption we can make safely. Otherwise, we keep judging each other as if we have the same opportunities in this life, which is the work of the enemy. As you've heard me say before, if the resources aren't available to all of us, it's hard to believe God requires any of us to follow these diet culture plans.

Diet Culture Has Hijacked Fasting as Well

Fasting is an age-old spiritual practice. We know it as the practice of abstaining from food for a specific period of time. I'm guessing there are some Jesus followers out there who have kept diet culture out of their fasting practices. I don't think I've met one of them, but I bet they're out there. For most of us, though, fasting from food can be a risky game. When I think of fasting in the days when Jesus walked this earth, I don't consider any sort of diet culture influence. Fasting in biblical times was typically practiced during times of urgent need, mourning, reflection, discernment, or atonement. There were certainly occasions when fasting happened in a communal context, but it was most often a private and intimate experience with God.

In the time of the early church, it was highly unlikely for a believer to fast in the hope that they would lose weight, and it's hard to imagine they would ask all their social followers to join them in that kind of fast. It's just a different situation today. Even with the best intentions at heart, fasting can foster diet culture desires instead of closeness to God. If diet culture wasn't our default lens, we might view fasting differently; however, like an out-of-context verse, fasting from food has become another potential tool for the enemy.

When churches require their staff and church members to fast from food together, they are likely unaware of how harmful fasting can be for some members. Church leaders can't possibly know about every member's developmental upbringing, medical history, or mental health status. The very act of mandating fasting removes the potential for intimacy in the process because it doesn't allow for an autonomous choice. Fasting of any kind is ultimately between you and God and is not intended to be a public display (see Matthew 6:16–18). If you choose to practice fasting from food, my prayer is that you will start from a fully fed state and you'll keep a close eye on ways that diet culture can sneak into your practice.

There are many ways today to get closer to God that have nothing to do with refraining from food or drink. When I think of what can stand in the way of my relationship with God, it isn't the eating of food. Many other things in our current culture—unrealistic task lists, social media, Netflix, ESPN, and doomscrolling, for example—interfere with our time, connection, and presence with God and with those we love. Dr. Bowers says that "fasting is less about food and more about a practice that draws our attention to our need for God." I'd go so far as to say that in our current times, being underfed, restricted, or engaged in purposeful dieting further diverts our attention from God.

You may feel the same way Jane did—that food was her idol. She would certainly say that her desire or "weakness" with regard to food made fasting something she believed she needed to practice. But what Jane didn't realize was that *her inability to fully feed herself regularly* led to feelings of want, specifically for foods she deemed "unhealthy." Jane had heard many pastors and teachers speak about food as a common distraction. If you grew up in diet culture, where food- and body-shaming messages are the default, it's the example to which you can relate. When diet culture has led us to believe that nourishment, something that is *required for living*, is wrong, it's no wonder we feel weak for desiring it.

Being underfed, restricted, or engaged in purposeful dieting further diverts our attention from God.

In my studies on fasting, I've uncovered no biblical commandment that requires it as a practice. Isaiah 58:6–7 reads as follows:

> Is not this the kind of fasting I have chosen:
> to loose the chains of injustice
>   and untie the cords of the yoke,
> to set the oppressed free
>   and break every yoke?
> Is it not to share your food with the hungry
>   and to provide the poor wanderer with shelter—
> when you see the naked, to clothe them,
>   and not to turn away from your own flesh
>   and blood?

When it comes to fasting, is food our yoke, or is our yoke our loyalty to a culture of injustice and oppression? I surely know which one we can live without.

If you were sitting in my office, we would be having these hard conversations together. If diet culture has enveloped you in lies about gluttony, temples, and fasting from food, we would talk through the lies one by one. We'd talk about the cultural context of fasting in ancient times when there were far fewer things to give up—food was a primary pleasure for everyday people in those times. If someone went without, it wasn't tied to a particular ingredient or to a weight goal. If someone honored their very real hunger, it wouldn't be called gluttony. We would bring truth to the many places where the lies of diet culture have snuck in, and I pray we'd be able to pull out the weeds of doubt once and for all.

All our current diets are wrapped in the spiritual shame of this world. I can't believe our good God wants us to be harmed by diet culture practices. We are already so deeply loved. We only have to accept God's love. It's the only ask. There is no earning this love. We have such a gracious God—a God so devoted, so gracious, so forgiving that nothing can separate us from that love. Not a meal. Not a snack. Not one single thing.

THE WORLD SAYS . . .

Your body and food intake are a
reflection of the temple of God.

THE WORD SAYS . . .

It is by grace you have been saved, through faith—
and this is not from yourselves, it is the gift of
God—not by works, so that no one can boast.

Ephesians 2:8–9

STEPPING AWAY FROM LIES

You made it! In part 1, we exposed the insidious nature of diet culture and the way it sneaks into our sacred and safe places. This unlearning and relearning can be difficult. The lies of this culture can be hard to uproot, especially if they've been planted in the soil of "safe" places.

- Think back to your first memories of the word *gluttony*. Was the term attributed to specific foods or bodies? What do you think about gluttony now?

- When you consider the full context of "your bodies are temples of the Holy Spirit," does it change how this verse lands on your heart?

- How can you move forward knowing that diet culture can be evicted from our reading of Scripture?

- Can you see how our current culture may interfere with ancient fasting practices?

- Review Ephesians 2:8–9. We are saved by God, not by our works. This gracious love is a gift we do not have to earn. As you recall the teachings of the chapters of part 1—exposing the lies of diet culture and how they keep us stuck—are you ready to move to truths? Let's go!

Dear Lord,

Open our hearts. Break them wide open. Help us have compassion for this journey. Give us the compassion for our own undoing—and compassion for others in the process. Lord, you made every part of us, even the parts this culture has told us to hate. Please open our eyes to help us see how diet culture eats away at the life you have given us. Give us eyes to see how this fixation on numbers, food, and bodies prevents us from seeing ourselves and our neighbors as you made us. Help us as we move to acceptance of the truth that our version of health on earth isn't required to receive God's love. Give us ears to hear the insidious whispers that hold us hostage in our own bodies. For you, O God, have given us freedom, which no person or thing can take from us. Don't let us ever forget that!

Lord, set us free from the numbers this world has taught us to count, for they are not a heavenly currency. Teach us to put in a rightful position our approach to eating and the movement of our bodies—not one that is greater than our connection with you or our relationships with your people. Remind us that you can use all things in this world for good. Give us a keen vision to see how this obsession with manipulating our bodies, as well as the bodies of others, can morph into another "wolf in sheep's clothing" in the blink of an eye. And, dearest Savior, open our eyes to fully see this deception in the "safe" places. The lies are cleverly wrapped in science and sound bites and recommended by those we've placed on pedestals of authority—our government authorities, doctors, teachers, pastors, and trusted influencers. Have we built body hatred and prejudice on a bed of lies? We plead for your wisdom.

Make our hearts open and ready for a stirring only you can bring about in a world so intent on measuring up and measuring us. Break down our understanding of health so we can rebuild something sacred. Help us disconnect today's cultural pairing of weight and worthiness, for we must realize that this lie did not come from you. Open our hearts so we may begin to see healing in situations where those who meant well have hurt us by wrapping your words around this world's food and body standards. Bring us to our knees, dear Lord. Breathe words of truth into our open hearts. Remind us that nothing on this earth—not our bodies, not our food, not our diagnoses, not our lack of abilities, not our sadness—can separate us from your all-encompassing love. This love is so great that it rises above and beyond all of our perceived deficiencies and doubts.

Mend us, dearest Lord. Empower us to hold each other with compassion. For to love you is to love one another—to love our neighbors as ourselves. Mend our hearts, Lord, as individuals and as communities. We pray this with our deepest love and gratitude.

AMEN.

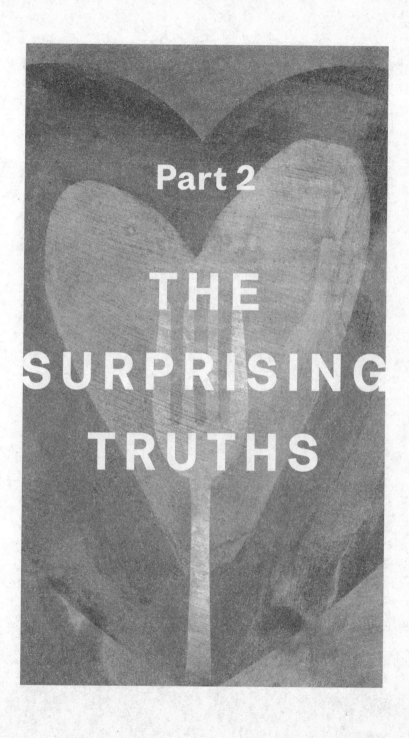

Part 2

THE
SURPRISING
TRUTHS

Truth #1

You Can Feed Yourself

> Nothing would be more tiresome than eating and drinking if God had not made them a pleasure as well as a necessity.
>
> **Voltaire**

We've come to the part of the book where you may expect that a dietitian will tell you exactly what to eat. But you don't need a dietitian for that. You may expect this is the spot for a chapter on "good" nutrition. But you don't need a nutrition chapter or yet another nutrition book with a cookie-cutter plan. If I were to throw at you a bunch of nutrition information and rules, I'd be erasing every word I've written so far. I'd be ignoring your lived experience, your privileges (or lack of), your medical history, your developmental history, your food traditions, your values, your abilities, and your food preferences.

Of course, I believe nutrition is important. I help people

with their nutritional strategies daily. But there is so much more to it. Giving nutrition advice without knowing a person's relevant nutritional, medical, and social history is a form of negligence. If I don't know you, giving you a specific nutrition plan can be harmful (hello, diet books and "health" influencers on social media). Handing out nutrition plans is not my job; rather, my job is to help you embrace the wisdom you already hold. I hope I can empower you to realize you have everything you need within you to feed yourself. At the same time, I'll help you dig up the very thing that years of living in diet culture has buried so deep—the confidence to feed yourself.

Imagine for just a moment that you're watching an infant who begins to feel hunger and gets fussy and cries. They will open their mouth and move their head toward food. They may get excited to see a bottle or pieces of food on their high chair tray. They have an innate sense that the milk or solid food will satisfy their underlying need. From the moment we are born, we have a sense of hunger and learn how to interact with our environment so that our need for nourishment will be met. We are truly born to eat. (I believe this so much that *Born to Eat* is the title of my first book.)

In diet culture, it's possible to watch this infant engage in honoring their body while completely forgetting that we too were once infants who had the very same skills. Babies often play with their feet, and toddlers get excited when they find their belly buttons. If you've watched them make these discoveries, it's easy to see how they demonstrate peace with their bodies. We also have this innate gift of knowing our bodies, but years of living in diet culture have made us afraid to trust this gift. It's there. I know it. I've never met a person who couldn't reconnect with their divine gift of attunement and body confidence. This reconnection won't look the same for everyone. But here is what is universally true: divesting from diet culture is a prerequisite.

We have a self-regulation system that is so close to perfect that only God could have designed it. Perhaps diet culture's most insidious "success" has been convincing us that we cannot trust ourselves. I bet you know where I'm going here, because I know you can see the lies now. You know that your body is good and trustworthy—or at least you're trying hard to believe and accept that truth.

> Perhaps diet culture's most insidious "success" has been **convincing** us that we cannot trust ourselves.

You Can Trust Your Body

Have you ever been watching a really good TV show at night and thought, *I really should go to bed*? The thought that you should go to bed may be prefaced by nodding off on the couch midway through an episode of your favorite show. You may not want to get up and do the bedtime routine that leads to tucking in for the night, but you don't question that your body is giving a signal that it's time for sleep. It's also likely that you don't second-guess your tongue when it feels dry and you decide you should drink some water. We trust these innate self-regulation signals. Sleepiness signals the need for rest. Thirst signals the need for hydration.

It's odd how we have no problem trusting specific signals our body gives us—like sleepiness, thirst, or the urge to go to the bathroom—but when we feel the signals of hunger, we batten down the hatches because the hurricane of "how can it be?" questions is getting ready to blow through. *But I just ate a few hours ago; how can this be? Since I had a big breakfast, shouldn't I skip lunch? How can I be hungry when it's not time to eat? Why do I eat so much?* Diet culture keeps us questioning our divine design. But the truth is that your body is wise. If you're hungry, you need to eat.

It wasn't always this way. You cried as a baby, ready to be fed, and you ran in from playing as a child, hungry as a hippo. You trusted your body. Doubt never crossed your mind. Thankfully, you can find that trust again.

Have you ever lost trust in someone and had to repair that relationship? The wound may have healed over and left a scar. It's possible this may be a chronic wound for you. The repairing starts with affirming that you value the relationship. In this case, the relationship is with your body. Losing trust in our bodies with regard to hunger and eating can feel like that—tightness where there should be flexibility, restriction where there should be abundance. The wound was inflicted by diet culture. And even though the harm that resulted can leave you afraid and unsure, healing is possible, especially when you're able to see that diet culture caused the wound, not your body.

Healing Begins with Feeding

The advice may sound quite simple, but when I tell my clients that healing typically begins with eating three meals a day, I get some crazy looks. This culture leads us to question whether we should put food in our bodies after not eating during the overnight hours. *Eating three meals and a couple of snacks each day is normal and appropriate.* And no, a coffee or granola bar does not constitute a meal—that's a nice snack.

Feeding our bodies adequately and consistently may be hard for the part of us still feeling wounded by diet culture, but it's the only way to heal. There's also a part of us that likely knows that skipping meals does not promote health. Affirming this part of us that desires freedom from diet culture will help us when feeding ourselves feels like a challenge. Feeding ourselves is never the wrong answer.

Eating regular meals and snacks may feel like a simple start. For others, it may be a very big challenge. I can tell you that the granola bar and coffee won't cut it, but only you know how much is enough, which is why I don't give canned nutrition plans. I don't live in your body. I am not the expert of your body. You are. Now, sometimes I have clients experiment with amounts of food. I say, "How did the eggs and toast feel for breakfast? How long did it keep you satisfied? If you were hungry two hours later, maybe you could try adding more and see how that feels. You could also add a midmorning snack." You are in charge of you.

> Eating three meals and a couple of snacks each day is **normal** and appropriate.

In all my years of practice, many clients have shared a consistent complaint: "I eat so well during the day, but then I get so hungry that I go off the rails at night." There hasn't been a time when this didn't translate to, "I tried to eat the way diet culture tells me to eat, which is too little for my body. It turns out I'm really hungry at night because I didn't eat enough during the day. That darn diet culture wound prevents me from truly nourishing and trusting my body. Then I feel awful—mentally and physically. Help!"

One of the most common issues for clients is getting enough food intake during the day (what I call front-loading), which can help protect afternoons and evenings from bouts of fierce and frantic hunger (like those experienced by Ricky, whom you met in the introduction). Eating breakfast, lunch, and a couple of snacks during the day before having dinner is normal. Diet culture has taught us that we should be existing on coffee, expensive supplements, and bits of lettuce—and that approach makes us question our very normal desire for food and the hunger that results during a day of eating too little. As I tell my clients, if we're not front-loading, we're back-loading. It's perfectly normal to eat several times during the day. We can trust our good and wise bodies.

Now, you may be thinking, *If I trust my body and eat regular meals and snacks, I'll gain weight.* Diet culture has planted the seeds of fear of weight change. Can your weight change? Sure, your weight may increase, decrease, or stay around the same range your entire adult life. Bodies change over the life span, particularly fed bodies. And it's unusual for them to drastically and permanently shrink. But you now know that your health and worth aren't tied to any numbers. When we're focused on "weight control," we're not able to focus on honoring the body's internal regulation system—the system we witness when an infant honors signs of hunger and eats until satisfied. We cannot honor the body and chase numbers at the same time. The two are simply incongruent.

In my office, there will be no stepping on that metal idol. We'll talk about the way you feel after eating more regularly and how you can plan to continue your journey with both familiar and new foods you may want to incorporate. You may be feeling more alert at work with adequate nourishment. You may be able to laugh more and engage in relationships with regular eating. Feeding yourself is a gift—to yourself and to everyone around you.

I Do Want to Warn You

Sadly, people stuck in diet culture don't understand people who are seeing the light and wanting to be free from it. My clients and I call this "swimming upstream." Although commenting on someone's food choices or body shape is incredibly rude and presumptuous, diet culture has led people to believe your body is their business. It is, unquestionably, *not*.

You may very well hear comments directed at your eating practices or choices—especially if you're eating consistently and adequately—as well as your appearance. Mature adults should know better than to cast judgments, but they don't always demonstrate sensitivity and grace. But we can set boundaries with others to protect ourselves. We can let people know that commenting on our food and bodies is not okay. In my home, I jokingly say I have a rule for guests: no food talk or body talk—and please leave by nine o'clock. Well, it's not actually a joke. Boundaries keep us safe and teach people what is okay and not okay. They also set guidelines for what's appropriate and not appropriate for little ears.

Although commenting on someone's food choices or body shape is incredibly **rude** and presumptuous, diet culture has led people to believe your body is their business. It is, unquestionably, *not*.

Getting reconnected with our internal regulation system can take work. I often help clients regulate their eating by pointing them to eating regular meals and snacks. Then I ask them to tune in to their bodies several times a day. "What does hunger feel like? Is it a gentle, empty feeling, or can you feel your stomach churning? Do you hear your stomach growling? Do you feel light-headed or hangry, or have a headache?" If so, they've gone too long without nourishment.

The goal is for you to feel confident when checking in with yourself. I hope that hunger becomes like a gentle tap on the shoulder rather than the all-too-common punch in the face. The more we tune in to ourselves during meals and snacks, the more confident we can become in our self-regulation system. The ability to sense fullness and satisfaction comes along with this practice as well. We may even get better at honoring our food preferences—what truly tastes good to us and what doesn't.

DOES SENSING BODILY CUES WORK THE SAME WAY FOR EVERYONE?

Some people, particularly those with a history of disordered eating, who are recovering from an eating disorder, or who are neurodivergent, may have a harder time with interoception, or the sensing of bodily cues. The struggle may feel like total preoccupation with a project so that no thought is given to eating, or it may feel like bouts of anxiety that mask the sensations of hunger or fullness. Some people are on medications that interfere with bodily attunement. It doesn't mean it's not possible to connect with your self-regulation system in some way. It just means it looks different, and that's okay. If this resonates with you, I strongly recommend working with a dietitian who understands intuitive eating and is experienced in supporting those with disordered eating or neurodivergence.

You Can Trust Food

With all the fearmongering about food and ingredients these days, it's not surprising we can worry ourselves sick over our food selection. Do we pick organic foods and low-ingredient crackers? What if we can't pronounce items on an ingredient list? Let me tell you how little all of that matters. Unless you have a medically diagnosed food allergy or intolerance from a physician who is board-certified in allergy and immunology—not just a report from unproven food sensitivity tests—overthinking these details can cause harm.[1] And how you spell or pronounce something on an ingredient list doesn't matter at all. That kind of concern reflects diet culture folklore.

Pick the food that is accessible to you and your family. Nourishing food encompasses all foods, including regional or cultural foods. If you grew up with traditional foods in your family, those foods are part of eating in a health-promoting way. Don't let anyone tell you any different. Stripping food heritage from our plates isn't about health; it's about discrimination.

If we banish the rules of diet culture, food is just food. Now, I'm not saying all foods are nutritionally equivalent. They're not, so eating a variety of foods is a good idea. But to eat in a way that keeps diet culture off our plates, foods need to be emotionally equal. That means the brownie that used to cause you worry can sit beside your chicken salad wrap and not freak you out because it's a brownie. It can also mean that the obligatory lunch salad can have toppings such as croutons, meat, and full-fat dressing. The brownie is food. The chicken salad wrap is food. The croutons are food. Food is food.

When food is just food, it can be emotionally equivalent. There's no good, bad, healthy, unhealthy, or otherwise. When food is food, there's no more, "Let me eat all the brownies now so I don't have to worry about them later." There's no more, "I can only eat salads because they're nutritionally superior," which often leaves us unfulfilled and longing for more, and may lead to bingeing later on. There's no more eating only this carefully prescribed amount of calories at lunch because it's the preplanned or allowable amount. God gave us taste buds, not oral calculators.

When we tell diet culture to get off our plates, we're left with just food. Food that we have every right to enjoy. Food with no label, like a juicy North Carolina tomato, and food with a long list of ingredients, like my beloved Cheez-It crackers. Food that brings us joy and celebration, and food that gets us through another day. God has blessed us with all of it.

Our Amazing Bodies Can Handle All the Foods

Our stomachs aren't fussing over ingredients. They're just digesting and putting that energy to work. Diet culture has taught us to fear and dissect every little bit of food. The enemy loves a good distraction, like laboring over a food label! We can stop micromanaging and worrying over every bite. Nothing in diet culture can do what our fearfully and wonderfully created bodies can—if we let them. And hear this: food is a basic need in life. Whether we sit in an office chair all day, chase after a kid, or hit the gym for a workout, our bodies need to be fed. Nourishment is not something we earn. Just imagine a tiny baby fussing for a bottle while we're thinking to ourselves, *They need to do some push-ups first.* Earning food is a nonsensical notion perpetuated by diet culture. We can let go of that idea, tune in to our bodies, and honor them by feeding them.

Of course, you're free to make food choices that make you

feel good. I love eating out, particularly at the pizza place up the street from my house. But if I were to eat there every day, I might long for more variety. (I'd also be broke.) So I may plan to eat there periodically and have other meals at home. You may want to add more fruits and a variety of vegetables to your meals. You can eat plant-based foods without giving up any other foods you like. Keeping frozen and canned fruits and veggies on hand can help add variety quickly and economically. Exploring seasonal options can be a fun activity if you have a farmers market near you.

IS IT ENOUGH?

Food security (having enough food and having quick access to it) is the necessary foundation for food freedom that leads to adequate, consistent, and pleasurable nourishment. I pray you have enough and have it consistently. Please don't forget that not everyone has food security. If you can help someone be more food secure, please do so. You may consider volunteering with or donating to a local food bank or organizations such as World Central Kitchen and Feeding America.

You may want to make some changes in your eating habits, like having a full and satisfying breakfast. That's great. I hope you feel nourished and energized as you start your day. Adding a breakfast meal may mean grabbing a pack of peanut butter crackers and a banana at a convenience store near work. Start with whatever works for you. And ignore the diet culture prophets who would shame you or disagree with your choice. They don't know you, nor do they have your genetics, lived experience, or budget. You are feeding yourself, not them.

You may not want to add or change anything about feeding yourself, and that's absolutely fine too. You don't owe anyone variety or vegetables. I just hope you have enough. What a radical act in this world—to feed yourself adequately in a culture that values restriction and control. Your life does not belong to diet culture. It is a gift to you from a good God. Please receive it. It's time to feed yourself and take back your life.

THE WORLD SAYS . . .

You don't need to feed yourself. Try
to get by on as little as possible.

THE WORD SAYS . . .

The angel of the LORD came back a second
time and touched [Elijah] and said, "Get up and
eat, for the journey is too much for you."

1 Kings 19:7

STEPPING INTO TRUTH

Our world can make us question the most basic form of self-care—feeding ourselves. It doesn't have to be that way.

- Consider the seeds about feeding yourself that were planted in your mind from an early age. Did those seeds grow into body confidence or body doubt? Were they tied to the way your body looked?

- How can you start to pull the weeds and disconnect the act of feeding your body from the worth or appearance of your body?

- What small steps can you take to propel yourself toward adequate and consistent nourishment?

- Would it be helpful to ask for support or talk to a friend about this journey? It is a journey, for sure, and it's also a revolution. Feeding yourself fully and pleasurably is an act of defiance against the enemy.

- Take a moment to reflect on 1 Kings 19:7. You may remember the story of Elijah fleeing from Queen Jezebel and hiding in the wilderness. When Elijah was sleeping, the angel of the Lord woke him up to give him something to eat in preparation for the journey and mission ahead of him. And so Elijah ate and was later empowered to feed others. What would it look like for you to get up and eat so you can be strengthened for the journey?

Truth #2

You Can Value Your Physical Health without Dieting

and i said to my body. softly.
'i want to be your friend.'
it took a long breath.
and replied
'i have been waiting my
whole life for this.'

Nayyirah Waheed, "Three"

Diet is a tricky word that has become synonymous with bodily restriction and a desire for weight loss. Once upon a time, the word *diet* simply meant a collection of the foods a person eats. These days, *diet* most often represents a collection of rules and restrictions that limit or control the body in some form or fashion.

Dieting, as We Know It Now, Is Not Required for Health

I am aware, painfully aware actually, of how countercultural it sounds to say that dieting is not required for health. But it's true. In my decades of helping people escape dieting and diet culture, not one person has said to me, "I have found health and happiness in restricting my body." It's usually the opposite, and they are sick and tired of chasing health through the latest diet trend.

When I was transitioning from being a weight-focused dietitian to a weight-neutral dietitian, I wasn't up front with people about the changes in my practice. I was worried if I said straight up, "I don't offer diets for weight loss," I'd lose clients. Then I realized that I was losing them because I wasn't forthcoming about my philosophy and process. Now when new clients reach out with the goal of working on their health through dieting, I try to be clear about what my approach will be.

An initial email message or phone conversation might go like this:

> Thanks for reaching out. I like to let my clients know that I do not focus on weight loss as a goal. It makes sense that weight is a concern for you in our diet-focused culture, yet evidence suggests that weight-loss dieting is not sustainable or health-promoting. I can help you focus on behaviors that feel good to you and will be health-promoting. It may or may not change your weight, but it can positively impact your health and relationship with food. Is this something you're interested in pursuing?

Almost every time, they respond with something like, "Yes,

I'm interested. I had no idea this type of practice was even an option."

With my new clients, I gather a complete history that includes things like their experience with food growing up, their food sufficiency, their beliefs about types of foods and bodies, and much more. When we meet for our initial session, I share that even though our culture and healthcare systems promote weight loss at every turn, pursuing weight loss does not promote health. We talk about how growing up in this culture can impact our adult habits and how, if desired, we can work on changing unhelpful behaviors or adding behaviors that feel good to them yet don't include dieting. Believe it or not, there are many ways to invest in our health without going on a diet.

Weight Is Not a Behavior

"Weight is not a behavior"—this is a statement I make often in my office. We've been led to believe it's possible to control our weight, but many factors influence our weight. While we can put a stop to certain behaviors—for example, smoking and excessive alcohol consumption—we can't change our body size and expect it to stay that way. Our divinely created bodies want to be what they were designed to be, regardless of cultural expectations.

Our divinely created bodies want to be what they were designed to be, regardless of cultural expectations.

Our genetics play a leading role in the size of our bodies, much like they do with regard to our height, skin, hair, and eye color.[1] Social and environmental factors also play a part (remember the social determinants of health and adverse childhood experiences). Does our nutrition play a role? Sure, a bit, but as I've mentioned before, it's nowhere near what we make it out to be. And don't forget, nutrition isn't dieting; nutrition, via the blessing of food, is what you *give* your body.

MY HEALTH PROVIDER SAID I NEED TO DIET TO LOSE WEIGHT FOR MY HEALTH

The evidence to date shows that weight-loss dieting promotes disordered eating, causes harm, and is primarily unsustainable. It is not health-promoting—just the opposite—and some researchers would even call it unethical.[2]

You and I know that weight isn't a behavior. Engaging in weight-neutral, health-promoting behaviors such as getting adequate sleep, eating consistently throughout the day, and moving our bodies offers health benefits like improved blood pressure, blood lipid levels, fitness levels, and mental health.[3] Sometimes people experience weight changes with behavior change, and sometimes they don't, and it isn't something anyone, including health professionals, can promise, predict, or control. If it feels like a safe request, ask your health provider for non-weight-based options or to give you the kind of advice they'd offer to a thin person.

Dr. Katja Rowell says, "I truly believe doctors who embrace a weight-neutral approach could have higher job satisfaction and be better at their jobs. I know their patients would benefit as well."[4]

So now what? We can talk now about behaviors we can control that may positively influence our health. Echoing what I typically say to my clients, let's start with your schedule. Ricky, whom you met in the introduction to this book, gave me a glimpse of his daily routine. I asked him to take me through his typical day, from the time he opens his eyes until he closes them. I often follow up with questions like, Do you have coffee or water, eat meals, grab snacks, drink other drinks, move your body, go to work? Do you eat meals with someone else or alone? Do you eat at your desk? Do you know what you're having for lunch or dinner, or do you usually decide in the moment? Do you have enough food? Are there foods you dislike? Are there foods you avoid? Why is that? I ask *a lot* of questions about the typical day.

This little exercise helps me get a feel for the pace and pressure of my clients' day-to-day lives. And if truth be told, we've all been a bit frantic lately, just like Ricky. We've forgotten to write self-care into our schedules, and it's not surprising. Diet culture seems to be a close cousin of hustle culture, and the grind just isn't healthy.

Remember Yourself in Your Schedule

It sounds a bit crazy because, hello, it's *your* schedule. But the first thing we work on in my office is the issue of looking out for yourself. Do you even have room to try the new behaviors you have in mind in your daily life? There will be no sitting outside eating a yummy lunch you packed when your break is spent blazing through emails to get to the next meeting. Some jobs are intense and inflexible, like when an employer dictates your specific work hours or you have strict shifts and regulations. But sometimes our schedules are crazy because we've allowed them to be crazy. That's the way my job was early in my career, especially when I started my own business. Then I realized the craziness resulted from my lack of boundaries around my time and achievement addictions (hello, hustle culture, and thank you, therapy). I realize this isn't the case for everyone, but sometimes we have more control over our daytime hours than we think.

We don't get medals for being overly busy or skipping meals in this life. We get ulcers, high blood pressure, anxiety, desperate hunger, and sleepless nights. When we take some time during the day to recharge and refuel, we can experience more instances of quality time both at work and outside of work. At some point, we have to reclaim small pieces of time during the day for self-care activities such as taking a mental break or having a meal away from our computers and phones. Remembering ourselves in our schedules is a health-promoting behavior.

How's Your Sleep?

The quality of sleep is usually the next topic we cover in a nutrition session. When we're exhausted, it's tough to make decisions, much less try out new behaviors. When I was in my nutrition program, we didn't talk about sleep in terms of how it could positively or negatively influence health. I don't remember studying it at all. Now research suggests that getting adequate sleep plays a crucial role in our overall health.

After we discuss your typical day, we'll consider your nighttime routine. I'll inquire about your screen time before bed or whether you have a wind-down habit. Then I'll ask you if you think you get enough sleep, because adequate rest matters a lot. Did you know that poor sleep is related to increased cardiovascular risk?[5] You can suck down all the kale smoothies in the world (if you like them), but it won't make up for not getting enough sleep. When we sleep poorly—the nights we fall asleep just fine but then wake up and have a hard time falling back to sleep—our risk for cardiovascular disease and cardiovascular events increases.[6]

I've had my share of sleepless nights. I think we all have

trouble sleeping sometimes. But when sleeplessness becomes a chronic concern, it's something we can work on as a health behavior. We can try more calming activities instead of using screens like our phones, computers, or televisions right before bed. The options might include reading a physical book, journaling about our day, praying, or practicing deep breathing.

Sometimes we can do all the things and still need help sleeping. One of my close friends has had trouble getting good sleep since she was a child. She remembers tossing and turning as a child, and she tells of other family members who struggled with sleep too. When she realized that her sleep was taking a toll on her mental and physical wellness despite her best efforts, she decided it was time for help. Her doctor was able to help her by using a variety of interventions. Asking for help with her sleep issues was a health-promoting behavior.

Have You Tried Joyful Movement?

Many of my clients have never heard of joyful movement. I think that's because so many of us grew up thinking exercise was for punishment (drop and give me ten push-ups!) or weight loss (feel the burn!). Those kinds of associations will suck the joy out of movement very quickly. But what if we viewed moving our bodies as something joyful? I discuss this concept with clients when movement is something they're interested in exploring.

It's important to note that not everyone has the same abilities. What may seem like an excellent option for one person may be outside the realm of possibility for another. Having the ability to move freely in our bodies without pain or physical limitations is a privilege. I try to keep this in mind and will often make referrals to physical therapists for safe adaptations and guidance.

FINDING HELP

Are you concerned about your safety or strength in movement? Physical therapists (PTs/DPTs) can help get us back on track after an injury or illness, but they can also assess strength and stability to help prevent injury. In my opinion, they're underutilized in this way. If you have the option and feel the need, ask your medical provider for a referral to a physical therapist.

When a client expresses interest in exploring movement options beyond what we see in the fitness sector of diet culture, a whole new world opens up. It's no longer about changing our bodies; it's about celebrating them. You may love walking, but the #noexcuses nonsense has made it seem insufficient. Listen, if something feels good to your body, it's not only enough; it's just right.

There is no wrong way to move your body unless it's to conform to diet culture. There are many options when we drop diet culture's expectations of what movement should look like. You may want to hike, bike, dance, walk, lift weights, do yoga, tend your garden, or do martial arts. These options can be fun while helping us improve our cardiometabolic fitness levels, which also reduces mortality risk at any body size.[7] The good news is that joyful movement, or the separation of weight-loss expectations from fitness, leads to better health, regardless of a person's body weight.[8]

> There is **no wrong way** to move your body unless it's to conform to diet culture.

Movement may not be joyful for many people, and that's okay. Sometimes we move for other reasons: "I want to get stronger, although I don't like weight training," or "I don't love walking, but it helps my mental health and sleeping pattern." Ricky didn't love the idea of going for walks, but he liked spending time with his wife—and she liked to take a walk after dinner. He walked for connection, knowing he got other benefits too. Finding joy in movement isn't a requirement, and it isn't always achievable. But we can still move in ways that help us meet goals and needs outside of the approaches of diet culture.

> If you've never experienced joy when it comes to exercise, then the phrase "joyful movement" may seem unrealistic. Try replacing it with "movement that has the ability to meet me where I'm at—on any given day; exercise that doesn't feel like punishment."
>
> Jamie Carbaugh, personal trainer and creator of Fit Ragamuffin

Many of my clients have found that before they could be successful in incorporating movement into their lives, they had to separate the idea of moving their bodies from weight change or calorie burning. In other words, they had to disengage from diet culture teachings and adopt a mindset shift in which they set intentions to participate in enjoyable movement to help them feel good and to promote overall health, not to pursue diet culture metrics. Such intentions can lead to more joyful and sustainable movement. We're taking back exercise through joyful movement, in whatever way that may look for us individually. And that is a health-promoting behavior!

=== THE WORLD SAYS . . . ===

Diet and exercise are the biggest
determinants of health.

=== THE WORD SAYS . . . ===

We know that if the earthly tent we live in is
destroyed, we have a building from God, an eternal
house in heaven, not built by human hands.

2 Corinthians 5:1

STEPPING INTO TRUTH

It can be hard to abandon diet culture's definition
of health, but it's not impossible. You may
recognize that sleep is a health factor you can
focus on, or you may find ways to move more
joyfully or purposely apart from the corruption
of diet culture. You can value your health
without engaging in diet culture! I'm so glad we
have the option and blessing of unlearning.

- How have you begun to disengage from our
  culture's view of health? Did you know there are
  so many other factors to focus on if you want to
  pursue health behaviors?

- Do you pencil in time for self-care in your
  schedule (for example, getting groceries,
  meeting up with a friend, going for a walk, or
  getting your meals and snacks in)?

- Is there a behavior you'd like to change that may improve your health?

- If you knew that your "right now" body wouldn't change and believed that it is a good body (and it is), what activities or health behaviors would you be willing to try? By trying new things, we may be better equipped to disconnect from the pursuit of weight loss and shift our focus away from the pursuit of diet culture goals.

- Think about 2 Corinthians 5:1. We may have a tent on this earth—our earthly body—but we belong to an eternal kingdom that this world's view of health can't touch. We can pursue health as our earthly abilities allow, but it is not a prerequisite for kingdom love. Reflect on this truth.

Pursuing Health Will Not Guarantee Health

Your body is just as good on the days you must rest as the days you can run. Your body is good on the days you groan, the days you grieve, and the days you get your whole to-do list done. No pills, no pain, no trauma, and no shame can take your worth away. Your weight, strength, sense of safety, and income might change, but your belovedness is here to stay.

K. J. Ramsey, Facebook post, September 15, 2022

I remember everything about that day. On the way to my appointment, I drove down Poplar Avenue, one of the main roads running through Memphis, Tennessee. I was thinking about the great time I'd had speaking at a women's ministry retreat over the weekend and the beautiful spring day. It was just a regular doctor's visit. I would go in—check, check, check, all good—and get back to the office. But that's not how it happened. My quick lunch break checkup turned into fear, monitors, IV fluids, and uncertainty. My view of health changed in an instant. Forty-two days later, I was discharged from the hospital.

During my time in the hospital, various medical professionals would come into my room, and inevitably it would come up that I was a dietitian. I recall that one nurse seemed very surprised that a dietitian, whom he assumed did all the "healthy" things, could end up in the hospital. Even though health doesn't have a particular look or job title, we often make assumptions about our neighbors and their health, as well as the way health is or isn't achieved. But let me tell you, no one gets a health pass in this life. No matter how many health behaviors or practices you have in place, no one gets a lifetime guarantee that protects them from illness or injury—not even health professionals.

After those long and scary days in the hospital, I entered a season of loss. Family and friends who'd had long lives died. Even though disease and sickness had chased them throughout their lifetimes, they had made it to old age. I was comforted that they had gone to heaven, but losing them was still hard. As the season progressed, I also lost too many young friends. Their youth and health practices didn't save them from cancer or heart complications. Losing them wasn't just hard; it was devastatingly eye-opening. It was a season of constant sorrow and reflection.

This World's View of Health Isn't Available to Everyone

A thin, "superfood"-filled body is no guarantee of anything. Diet culture is largely to blame for our faulty belief that our health behaviors will inevitably lead to good health and longevity. Do health behaviors help? Sure. Do they prevent all the ailments? No. Our culture's false beliefs about "healthy" living have left us with a general lack of respect for the diverse lives we lead and bodies we inhabit. We want to feel in control of our health and our lives, which makes sense. But our false sense of control via dieting, "superfood" consumption, and food rules doesn't help.

I'm not saying you shouldn't engage in health behaviors. Please pursue health in ways that are important and accessible to you. But remember, there are no guarantees, and health looks different for everyone. Even though our health and medical communities try hard to tell us what health should look like, health cannot be defined by policy. Our bodies and our genetics don't care about policies. Your definition of what health will look like in your life is determined by you as an individual. And most likely it will not look like your neighbor's health.

> Our culture's false beliefs about **"healthy"** living have left us with a general lack of respect for the diverse lives we lead and bodies we inhabit.

Health encompasses much more than being physically well. Being physically well isn't an option for everyone, but you can pursue whatever your own definition of health entails. Do you remember Teri? She determined that health for her was staying in recovery. That meant following up with a weight-neutral doctor, eating three meals and some snacks daily, cutting off her shows by 9:00 p.m., getting adequate sleep, and spending time walking with a friend. When she engaged in these behaviors, she felt she was supporting health in a way that made sense to her. She knew the scale and BMI talk had only harmed her health in the past, so she decided to leave them out of her own definition. Teri also limited her time on social media and budgeted time and money to see her therapist every other week. Not only did defining health for herself help her feel a lot better, but her blood pressure readings and lab results also improved.

ARE "SUPERFOODS" A CURE-ALL?

The answer to the question, "Are superfoods a cure-all?" can be given in one word: No. The word *super-food* is a marketing term. We often see these foods tied to health-related claims about disease prevention and longevity. These foods tend to be fruits or vegetables that have emerged in diet culture with a health halo based on food and diet trends. Many have long been used as staple ingredients in other countries and cultures but now come with a new price tag. Eat them if you like them, but don't be fooled into thinking that a superfood label is a health guarantee.

Nicole, who was chronically counting calories, also realized she could define health for own body. After spending time in therapy for her anxiety, which set her up well for chronic calorie counting, Nicole decided that medication would be an aspect of her definition of health. When she took her medicine, she felt less worried about meeting everyone else's expectations, which improved her life. Health for Nicole also meant saying yes to less. She had overcommitted to extra projects at work and at church, which kept her from quality time with family and friends—the connections that made her feel well. Nicole wasn't free of medical diagnoses, and her weight had increased to heal her body after years of restriction. And she felt better than she ever had in her adult life. Her overall health, as it turned out, got better when she took weight and calories out of her definition.

If you remember the social determinants of health (SDOH) from chapter 4, you know just how multifaceted a person's health can be. As you determine what health will look like for you, consider the many variables that influence your own definition.

Such things as finances, access to healthcare, and physical abilities, which are benefits not everyone has, can determine how we pursue health or engage in health behaviors. Let's grow in our awareness of how these variables may influence our health and the health of our neighbors.

You May Be a Person with Wealth

Being wealthy may afford us things like gym memberships, different foods, nutritional supplements, or even workout equipment in our home, which are all fine things to invest in if we choose them, but they aren't options for everyone. If we're working multiple jobs to pay our day-to-day bills, we may not have money to spend on nutritional variety or gym memberships. Sometimes we forget and assume others can make the same choices with regard to health.

In most cases, wealth allows us adequate access to healthcare. If we have health insurance or are able to be self-insured, we can likely make preventative medicine appointments such as annual physicals, dental cleanings, and blood work as needed. Engaging in these appointments is a positive health behavior. However, it's a different story if we don't have access to healthcare, have trouble

> Equally damaging [to our expectations that all bodies should conform to our standards] is our insistence that all bodies should be healthy. **Health** is not a state we owe the world. We are not less valuable, worthy, or lovable because we are not healthy. Lastly, there is no standard of health that is achievable for all bodies.
>
> Sonya Renee Taylor,
> *The Body Is Not an Apology*

making or getting to appointments, or live where these medical options aren't near our home. Health isn't a simple choice, but it tends to be more accessible for those with wealth.

You May Be a Person with Time

Having a flexible schedule lends itself well to engaging in health behaviors. Although I'm often frustrated with the scheduling process for healthcare appointments, I have time or can make time in my schedule to tend to a medical concern. My clients have taught me that not everyone has the luxury of time, particularly when someone has a job that requires them to be on the clock at specific times. Taking time off may mean less pay, and less pay may mean a person can't afford the prescriptions they need or the food they need or want.

Having time in our schedule also allows for other health behaviors to take place. With flexibility, we may be able to shop for groceries more frequently, get in some joyful movement, and even prepare a few extra meals for a busy week. Having open pockets of time is an underrecognized health variable. We all have the same amount of time in a day or a week, but not everyone has the same options for how to use that time.

> We all have the same amount of time in a day or a week, but not everyone has the **same options** for how to use that time.

You May Be a Person with an Able Body

A couple of years ago, I tore my hamstring and had a lot of pain and limited mobility. Sitting in the car was hard. Going for a walk was hard. It took a very long time for the injury to heal. While I was hurting and healing, I learned a vital lesson. I had never acknowledged the benefits my able body allowed me. Being able to walk pain-free and without mobility devices my entire life has permitted me to navigate things like fitness, travel, and grocery aisles, to name just a few, without concern. This isn't always the case for those with a disability or chronic disease.

Everyone on this planet was created on purpose, made in the image of God and worthy of pursuing health however they see fit, no matter how their body moves or doesn't move. Having the ability to move freely in our bodies does allow certain advantages in terms of health and health behaviors. This is one of the many reasons we can't allow diet culture to define health for us—it discriminates and leaves so many image bearers out of the equation.

You May Be a Person with Inside Information

Some people have the option to have this information, and some do not. You may be genetically predisposed to certain diseases in your lifetime. An example of this may be knowing that you're at higher risk for certain types of cancer because you've had genetic testing. Based on the results of these tests, you may or may not be able to take action to reduce the chances of getting that type of cancer down the road.

I've worked with people who knew that they had a higher risk for certain cancers and had preventative treatments to decrease their risk of a later diagnosis. Others have received information suggesting they'd likely encounter a scary disease at some point in their future. However, this information led to drastically changed eating habits, eating disorders, and malnutrition. The fearmongering around health risks, food choices, and death can make any of us take it too far. We can have information about our family histories, genetic risk factors, and disease states without letting it take hold of us.

Pursue Health, but Keep a Loose Grip

Like scales, tracker apps, and wearables, we can make anything an idol, even the pursuit of health. I think we can pursue health behaviors that align with our values as long as we don't hold on too tight. When I think about my health behaviors, I check myself to see if they align with my values. My values include lifelong learning, connection with others, and strength. Walking with my friends and hiking with my family support my value of connection. Cooking meals with my family and sitting with my friends at church also support that value. Sometimes I listen to books or podcasts while out walking (my clients and I call it "pod-alking"). These behaviors align with my value of lifelong learning. I like to lift weights and have daily devotional or God time. Both of these activities support my value of strength.

I often ask clients to think about their own values in my office. This is something I discussed with Teri and Nicole. They realized that trying to achieve a health policy view of health wasn't helpful for them. They needed to define it on their terms with their values. Sometimes when we're having this conversation, I share my own values as an example. Values can often be supported by many different behaviors, especially during

We can make anything an idol, even the pursuit of health.

different seasons of our lives. When I spent time in the hospital, my overall view of health had to change. When I hurt my leg, my idea of health behaviors had to change. Our views of health and our health behaviors will change throughout our lives because our bodies and circumstances will, inevitably, change.

Today, I consider myself relatively healthy. Do I have health concerns? Yes. Do I engage in health behaviors that feel good to me? Yes. Do I keep a loose grip? You bet I do, because I know I may need to redefine health again. This worldly view of health could be gone at any moment. And it is not offered to everyone.

There is beauty in the loose grip. There is also less pressure. I remember a pastor's story about his car breaking down and how he started getting very angry about the car and his situation. He reminded us through the story that it is all God's, everything, including us. Aren't we so much more important to God than a broken-down car? You bet we are, and our earthly level of health cannot change that fact. We may not have a guarantee of health in this life, but we have an ultimate promise that we will not be alone, no matter where our health journey leads us. Go ahead, loosen your grip.

THE WORLD SAYS . . .
Health is achievable through
hard work and willpower.

THE WORD SAYS . . .
"For I know the plans I have for you," declares
the Lord, "plans to prosper you and not to harm
you, plans to give you hope and a future."
Jeremiah 29:11

STEPPING INTO TRUTH

Thinking about our health can be daunting at times. I'm curious—have you been trying to measure up to a worldly policy view of health? It's okay. I have as well. And at times I fall back into the blaming and shaming we've learned from diet culture.

- Are you ready to let go of some of those earthly diet culture–related health goals? How would you now define health?

- Have you thought about how your health behaviors may align or not align with your values?

- What might your health behaviors look like knowing what you know now?

- Have you considered variables like time, wealth, information, and an able body as health benefits before? Do you have some of those benefits? Are there benefits you don't have?

- Armed with this information, can you more easily have compassion for a neighbor worried about their health and refrain from making assumptions about their situation?

- How might you begin to loosen your grip on the worldly view of health?

- Think about Jeremiah 29:11. God knows everything about our lives—the health concerns, the waiting-for-the-test fears, the possible diagnosis, and the treatment options. Yet God's plans are to prosper us and not to harm us. There is hope and a future; not one piece of it is tied to this world's view of health.

Truth #4

Mental Health Is Vital to Overall Health and Well-Being

Being able to feel safe with other people is probably the single most important aspect of mental health; safe connections are fundamental to meaningful and satisfying lives.

Bessel A. van der Kolk, psychiatrist and author of *The Body Keeps the Score*

Danielle moved around a lot. Her family moved to a new state every couple of years for better job opportunities and health-care options. She'd find a new place to live, get everyone ready to go, pack the moving truck, and head toward a new town. This last move hit her harder than the others. Her neighborhood had become so unsafe that she'd lie awake, fearing for her children's safety. Her anxiety was on high alert, and sleepless nights became her new norm.

I've had the tremendous privilege of working with Danielle off and on for more than a decade. She'd suffered from health anxiety, chronic restriction, and overexercise. Although she'd been feeding herself well without food rules, her anxiety triggered restrictive thoughts about her food and body. This time, she recognized the parts of her that needed attention instead of acting on the urge to restrict. She realized that her stress and anxiety related to another move were triggers that made her overfocus on food or her body.

For the first time in years, Danielle saw how her mental health played a role in her physical health. She understood that her underlying anxiety, coupled with some unhelpful advice from a previous healthcare provider, had been the perfect storm for many years. She now knew that her food and body didn't need to change. It was time to concentrate on her mental health and emotional well-being.

Our Mental Health Plays a Significant Role in Our Overall Well-Being

It's unlikely we'll live stress-free in this fallen culture of diet and hustle, but we must acknowledge the way our mental health influences our physical health and relationships. We cannot ignore stress and anxiety or act like they only hurt "those weak people." Mental illness can impact anyone. If any type of health is wealth, it is your mental health. We must be open to seeking and receiving help.

The very same pastor who told the story of the broken-down car also talked about caring for our psychological well-being. The storytelling pastor spoke about going to therapy and jokingly said, "I used to worry about the people who went to therapy; now I worry about the people who don't!" It's essential for us to recognize that God has given us many options for help in this world. The Bible is our foundation as believers, but God has provided us with wonderful helpers in this life as well, such as therapists and, when needed, medication.

Almost 53 million Americans have a mental illness—that's about one out of every five people.[1] There are many types of mental illnesses, but two of the most common are depression and anxiety. As we've crawled out of a worldwide pandemic, mental health concerns associated with loneliness are on the rise.[2] Even before the pandemic, loneliness was a common reason many of my clients suffered from eating concerns. It makes so much sense to me now, knowing that we humans are designed for connection with others.

Connection via Positive Relationships Reduces Mortality Risk

We spend a lot of time talking about factors such as smoking, alcohol use, physical inactivity, and body weight in our health system, mainly in terms of the way they may increase the risk of death. I agree that smoking and alcohol abuse aren't good for us. I also think moving our bodies in joyful, accessible ways is important. But did you know that having good relationships has roughly the same influence on mortality risk as quitting smoking or drinking, and *even more* than movement or body weight?[3] It's true. Our social relationships can be very beneficial to our mental and physical health. And I'm not talking about social media connections. I'm talking about the real, face-to-face, human kind.

What we need to be talking about at health visits is

connection, not dieting or weight loss. We spend way too much time talking about things we have little control over. What if we could focus on something that costs so little and helps so much—namely, relationships? We must start having these conversations, because poor relationships due to loneliness and social isolation are associated with an increased risk (of about 30 percent) of developing coronary heart disease or having a stroke.[4] And that was before the COVID-19 pandemic. We are wired for connection. God made us that way, and science confirms it.

We've All Been a Bit More Anxious Lately

It's no surprise that experiencing a pandemic and multiple lockdowns had a significant impact on our anxiety levels. Many of us dealt with anxiety long before COVID-19 was a part of our vocabulary, and our anxiety symptoms escalated once the pandemic erupted. It definitely didn't help, especially for those who experienced increased anxiety symptoms due to post-COVID-19 syndrome.[5] Some of us may not even realize we have anxiety. We may just think that we get flushed and our heart races from time to time for no apparent reason. Have you ever had to run to the bathroom before participating in a big event? Thanks a lot, nerves!

Anxiety doesn't just hang out in the brain. It can wreak havoc in the whole body.

Anxiety doesn't just hang out in the brain. It can wreak havoc in the whole body. It's not unusual for me to be working with a client whose reason for seeking nutritional guidance is stomach pain and gastrointestinal issues. By the time they land in my office, they've tried a gazillion dietary changes to help reduce their symptoms. Most of the time, the issue isn't the food—aside from the fact that now they've become very restricted in their eating. The problem is often how their anxiety plays out in their bodies.

Neurotransmitters are chemical messengers of the central nervous system that send information throughout the body—sort of like little internal text messages sent from your brain to other parts of the body to get them ready for some type of action. My clients and I often discuss how these neurotransmitters may act in the gastrointestinal tract. Clients may report feeling nauseated, weirdly full, or bloated or needing to get to the bathroom immediately. Sometimes these neurotransmitters send messages that say, *I'm scared*, or *I'm in danger*, even when there is no clear reason for alarm.

Having these symptoms can be scary and uncomfortable, and we desperately want relief. Food elimination tends to be the first line of defense—*Okay, it's gotta be my food, so no more of this or that.* We've been programmed in diet culture to put the blame on food first for every possible ailment, but that's not usually the answer. In many cases, restriction and undereating, or low energy availability, make the problem even worse. Yes, some people have legitimate food allergies or diseases (like celiac disease) that need to be managed by eliminating certain foods, but I'm talking here about the far more common issue of unnoticed anxiety symptoms that cause physical distress.

If a client describes struggling with anxiety and food elimination, I will refer them to a therapist and on occasion a psychiatrist. We then can work as a team to help get their anxiety symptoms managed while getting them back to normal and adequate eating. When we have more options to manage anxiety, cope with stress, or process old wounds, the symptoms we tend to blame on food can often subside.

Depression and Anxiety Can Impact Anyone

After I graduated from college, I got married, moved to another state, and started a new job—all in the span of a few months. It was a happy and exciting time but also a new, uncertain, and stressful time. I was talking to one of my friends one day who just happened to be a therapist, and she said, "Leslie, I think you're depressed." That wasn't something I thought could be a problem because I was well versed in how to suck it up and keep moving. If that's what you've also learned, let me suggest that it is *not* a good strategy.

My therapist buddy told me it made sense that I was struggling because I had many risk factors, including a family history of depression, significant life changes, and a load of stress. She painted a picture of how I felt and gave it a name. It was *depression*.

RISK FACTORS FOR DEVELOPING DEPRESSION

- Previous experience of depression
- Family history of depression
- Major life transitions or changes
- Trauma or extreme stress
- Certain medications and physical illnesses

Depression isn't a choice. It is caused by a combination of genetic, biological, psychological, and environmental factors.[6] If you think you might be suffering from depression, please make an appointment with a medical or mental health professional. You can feel better. I know. I've been there.

Being a Christian doesn't guarantee we'll be free of earthly problems like depression or anxiety, but let me tell you, our faith can help us cope with our struggles. I've battled depression and anxiety (like millions of other Americans) off and on throughout my entire adult life. It would be harder if I didn't have a solid understanding of grace in my heart. I'm also fortunate to have been a part of Christian congregations that have acknowledged that God gave us not only the Word to guide us but also one another to form supportive connections, including fellow believers as well as helping professionals and support groups.

I know more people who have suffered from mental health issues than people who haven't. And praise the Lord, there are things we can do on this side of heaven to feel better— one of which is prayer. Spending time frequently in prayer seems to be a useful strategy for improving overall mental health.[7] Some research suggests that those who have a regular habit of prayer are more optimistic and have better coping strategies, in addition to experiencing less depression and anxiety.[8] If I had heard this when I was a baby Christian, I would have felt a lot of pressure to get prayer "right." But I now know there's not a right or wrong way to connect with God.

As I learned more about prayer, I realized it's really just a dialogue with God in my mind. One of my favorite pastors taught me that it's like a bullet list you just read off in your mind

> One of the great tragedies of depression is the isolation and shame people carry as a result. We need communities of faith that normalize depression. **Life is hard.** At some point we break. Depression is not a sign of weak faith. It's a sign that we are human and in need of support.
>
> Rich Villodas, Twitter post, September 6, 2022, 9:01 p.m.

and send to God. I often just chat with God in my head—and that's my prayer. If you don't know what to say, that's okay too. The Holy Spirit prays on our behalf when we don't have the words or strength (Romans 8:26–27). Being silent in God's presence is prayer. Listening quietly is prayer. Prayer can be fancy too, if that's what you like, but I don't think God cares which technique we choose. Just being in God's presence can help our mental health.

Sometimes the answer to those prayers comes in the form of helpers—a referral to a therapist, psychiatrist, or family physician, or a prescription for medication. Few things in my life have been more effective than talking through my thoughts and concerns with a therapist. It's a wonderful feeling to have an unbiased human being in your corner who is committed to helping you figure out how to navigate this world and live resiliently in it. Sometimes it's enough, and sometimes it's not. At times we may need medication as well. As my dear neighbor used to say, "Better living through chemistry, honey." *God has given us all the helpers.*

Movement tends to be useful in improving our mental health as well. When we're feeling down, the last thing we may want to do is go for a walk or to a workout class at the gym. This kind of movement might not be particularly joyful at first, but when we know we may well feel better afterward, we learn from experience that the joy, or mental boost, can come after the moving.

In addition to getting adequate sleep, taking in enough nourishment, and seeing a helping professional, my client Danielle found movement to be a supportive strategy for decreasing her stress level. Research supports this approach as well. Studies suggest that exercises such as aerobic activity, weight training, and yoga may help those with depression and anxiety feel better.[9]

It can also be very helpful to take a break from social media. Many of my clients take pauses from scrolling to benefit their mental health. It's simply not the type of connection that can ultimately heal us. One recent study suggests that even a one-week break from social media platforms can significantly improve a person's sense of well-being.[10] Just one week—imagine what a longer pause could feel like.

If we think about all the things that impact our psychological health, a central theme emerges. That theme is connection.

Our mental health plays a critical role in our overall physical health and well-being. If we think about all the things that impact our psychological health, a central theme emerges. That theme is connection. We are connected to each other as Christians, friends, family, neighbors, or helpers. We are wired for connection on purpose. When we find ourselves disconnected or isolated, it's probably time to seek help and fellowship.

THE WORLD SAYS . . .

Suck it up and keep moving.

THE WORD SAYS . . .

When anxiety was great within me,
your consolation brought me joy.

Psalm 94:19

STEPPING INTO TRUTH

I don't know what it was like growing up in your home, but in my home we didn't talk about stress, anxiety, depression, or mental illness.

- Was your experience similar to or different from mine? In what ways?

- Have you ever experienced the symptoms described in this chapter? You know I have, and I'm so glad we're talking about mental health. It's an essential factor in our overall health.

- Are you open to seeking help if you need it? You don't have to be in crisis to talk to a helping professional. In fact, given the challenges regarding access to care and possible delays in obtaining appointments, it's better not to wait.

- Can you see how connecting with others is imperative to your health and well-being? Is this something you'd like to work on? If so, how can you plan to pursue more connection with others?

- Take a moment to reflect on Psalm 94:19. Notice the verse reads *when* anxiety is great within us, not *if* anxiety is great within us. The stressors of this world will affect us, but God will give us consolation and joy. Let's not forget that God often does this through relationships and the guidance of helpers.

Truth #5

You Owe No One a Number on a Scale

> Your body is an instrument, not an ornament.
>
> **Lexie and Lindsay Kite, PhDs, creators of Beauty**
> **Redefined and authors of *More Than a Body***

Have you ever gotten the feeling that the person you're with has something really big weighing on their mind? That's the way it was for me when Crystal came to my office for her session. I'd been working with her long enough to know that her demeanor that day wasn't her norm. I got the sense that something was off.

When I asked her what was going on, Crystal stood up and said, "Do I have time to run home and come back? I'd like to give you something." The hour was hers, so I nodded and she walked out my office door. Fifteen minutes later, she walked back into my office with her scale and said, "I'm done with this!" As she put it on my table, I noticed she'd written on it with a black marker, "I choose to keep my power. So long, scale.

It's over!" And that was that! She was done letting that hunk of metal take her power and energy.

For the rest of the session, we talked about what led her to that moment of rejection of the scale. After years of allowing it to dictate her food intake and happiness, she'd had enough. It took up too much space in her heart and on her bathroom floor. She realized it had kept her from experiencing pleasure, honoring her body, and nurturing other connections in her life. She wasn't going to give one more moment of power to this idol of diet culture. It was time to gain freedom, to declare that she didn't owe anyone a number on that piece of metal. I still have her scale on the shelf in my home office as a great reminder that even though the enemy's arrows can be sneaky and swift, we *can* see them, evade them, and find freedom.

The Weight of This World Isn't Helping Us

Our weight has no bearing on our worthiness and very little to do with our health. God does not ask us to measure up by stepping on a scale. As our culture created a false hierarchy of bodies and sizes, many Christians started to believe their bodies were measures of goodness—a belief that couldn't be further from the truth.

It's worth noting that there isn't a single example of using a scale to measure bodies in the Bible. The scales most commonly mentioned in the Bible were the kind you find on fish, not the kind that weighs people or measures their worth. In Job 6:2, Job cries out for scales to measure his misery (maybe that's a little diet culture foreshadowing). There is no biblical example of attaching our value to a number on a scale, not even for the sake of a person's so-called health.

Sarah grew up in a very religious home. Her family was

loving, but they tied worth to her weight, which was the reason she became one of my clients. She had left her job to seek treatment for her eating disorder that had been fueled over time by her obsession with weight. Treatment was a long and hard road for her. She wanted her family's support, but they refused to disconnect her weight from her worth. When Sarah tried to tell her family that she needed to let go of weight monitoring to facilitate her healing, they simply couldn't understand this way of thinking.

Sarah's family had enfolded diet culture into their faith, and those false roots had grown deep in her soul and become her inner critic, leading ultimately to her eating disorder. Changing the way she was eating—from not having enough food to fully feeding herself and being able to live a full life—meant weight gain. To her parents, particularly her father, it meant failure, and she was heartbroken.

But as Sarah and I worked together, she started to realize that her experience had nothing to do with her faith; it was tied to generational trauma. I shared with her a glimpse of a God who resembled the God she had learned about as she was growing up, but one who accepted her as she was, no strings attached. The only God I know is one who is filled with grace and unconditional love.

As the weeks passed, we talked about God and how to care for a divinely made body, acceptable as it is in every respect. We talked about Jesus and the greatest love of all—a love so great that no number on any scale can change it. She realized that her hyperfocus on the scale kept her body restricted while affecting the way she used her voice and purpose.

One day, Sarah brought to our session a drawing of a brilliantly colored fish. Her therapist and I had asked her to journal about the ways her focus on the scale had taken so much of her time, attention, and ability to experience a full life. The magnificent fish seemed to be smiling in her picture, and the caption read, "Scales are for fish, not humans!" And just as Crystal did, Sarah took back her power and her voice—and you can too.

You owe no one a number on a scale, and you don't even owe it to yourself. If you think you do, take a moment right now to reflect on how that thought got planted in your mind. It sounds a lot like "new year, new you" or "summer body" language to me. Diet culture planted that seed. We live in a world obsessed with numbers and thinness, so it's pretty normal to fall victim to that way of thinking. We all want to feel like we belong, but listen, you already belong, just as you are. You already belong to the kingdom of God. You do not owe this world a number!

You don't owe a number on a scale to your partner either. If we can point to one aspect of diet culture that breaks relationships, it's objectification—viewing a human as made up of parts that need to be perfected in order to be desired. It leads us to pick apart ourselves and others (legs too big, boobs too small, arms not muscular enough, skin too wrinkly, and so forth). This objectification only leads to turmoil because God made human bodies to change and evolve over the course of our lives. Diet culture is the culprit, teaching us to expect others to look a certain way, even if it's not real or achievable. We take the false idols we've grown up with—the filtered photos in magazines, the images of social media, and the disordered practices in our circles—and hold our partners to unreachable standards.

You may even find so-called "Christian" books and articles

You owe no one a number on a scale.

that sanctify objectifying bodies, spreading the message that it's okay to require a "trophy" of a partner. Sadly, this is an example of objectification wrapped in a Bible verse. I've heard preachers give sermons about this, blatantly ignoring the teachings of Jesus' unconditional love. This message destroys intimacy and ultimately relationships, which crumble under the weight and harm of diet culture's lies and objectification while the enemy laughs. Objectification of bodies is oppression. The Jesus I know will never stand for the oppression of any image bearer's body.

As long as we focus on a number on a scale, we'll be disconnected from our true selves—a disconnect that can derail deep relationships with others, impede understanding of our bodies' signal, and spoil their enjoyment of delicious food. Because of diet culture, we have a troubled relationship with the scale and a mythical number rather than a loving relationship with our bodies and food. As we objectify ourselves, we deny our own divine design, and very likely the divine design of others, which in the end hinders us from having an uninhibited relationship with God as well.

It's not just partners who suffer. The impact also trickles down to children. Think about Sarah and the fact that her father was obsessed with her appearance and her

> **I sometimes wish men were leading this conversation, and with repentance, because they've been complicit in the cultural movement to hold women to the lie that they have to meet certain standards of beauty in order to make an impact for the Lord.**
>
> Jess Connolly, *Breaking Free from Body Shame*

"ideal" weight. Although diet culture pushes us to believe that health has a certain look to it (it doesn't), Sarah's experience in childhood was not about love and health. It was about objectifying the female body to please a male gaze. Her father taught her that her body was something to be viewed, no matter how much disordered micromanaging and harmful obsession it took. Growing up, Sarah watched as her mother barely fed herself and overexercised to keep her father's harsh words at bay and to avoid emotional neglect and disapproving glares. Sarah's future had been played out in front of her.

Her brother was watching as well, learning that one day he could hold a spouse to harmful standards. What a misrepresentation of God's purpose for their lives and future loving partnerships! This approach is surely not a reflection of the way Christ loved the church or his people. The church is a community of hearts and souls who love God and each other. No numbers or particular appearances are needed to please Jesus.

How misguided we've been to let these lies be planted in young minds and grow into thorny vines that strangle generations of relationships! I'm not sure that humans are fully capable of unconditional love on this earth, but we have to try. You owe *no one* a number on a scale. No one owes one to you either.

Remember, the weight check and possible unsolicited diet advice are the main reasons people who need and want to receive medical care skip going to the doctor. The obligatory weight check is a part of the patient's path to the exam room, but it is a thoughtless routine rather than a medical necessity. In the few cases when a weight check is needed—for dosing certain medicines, taking growth measurements for children and pregnancy, or tracking illnesses that may cause fluid retention—the check can be done blindly (the patient steps on the scale backward), and the numbers don't always require a discussion.

I often skip weight checks at my own medical visits. Sometimes I get pushback, and sometimes I don't. My many privileges play a role here. I have the option to contact a new medical professional if I don't like how their office treats me, and my body size is rarely to blame for my ailments. This isn't the case for everyone, particularly those living in larger bodies who regularly face weight bias or those who are afraid they'll be refused care otherwise. The more that those who feel safe say, "No, thank you," to the weight check— standing against this unnecessary tradition—the safer medical spaces will become for all bodies.

Isn't Weight a Vital Sign?

Is weight a vital sign? The primary answer is no. Weight checks are customary but typically unnecessary. If you had a telemedicine appointment with a medical provider during the pandemic, a weight check couldn't be taken. You may have even received problem-focused care instead of weight-focused care. Now that office visits have resumed, we're back to the same old routine. And whether or not you want weight loss, diet, or exercise advice, you (or your insurance) can be billed for it.

In most cases, a weight check is unwarranted. It is needed when a physician prescribes a medication that involves weight-based dosing—for example, in cases of preparing anesthesia (nobody wants the medical team guessing on the correct dosage!). Those with an illness that causes fluid shifts and retention may need weight checks to determine a course of treatment. In these cases, the weight *change* is the vital sign, not the weight itself.

When I speak on this topic, often someone asks whether weight change is a vital sign of health and wonders whether we should get our weight checked just to be sure that everything is okay. Doing so might be warranted if we didn't receive healthcare in a weight-biased system. However, we do live in an incredibly weight-biased culture. It's possible that if someone lost weight over time due to an underlying illness, a provider might congratulate them on the change. On the flip side, if someone experienced significant and unexplained weight gain, it's possible they'd be offered diet and exercise advice instead of further inquiry or testing.

Sadly, I've seen this type of weight stigma happen with my clients time and time again. While it isn't the case for everyone, in general, the more we abstain from unnecessary weight checks, the greater the potential to have helpful conversations with our health providers about when such checks are warranted for our care.

Suppose you think this is all nonsense (which I get—I've been there). Let me ask you this: Has our war on ob*sity or culturally nonconforming bodies "worked"? The answer is no. We worship the gods of false health and weight. The "health" of this nation is worse than ever, not because people fail at weight loss but because weight-loss attempts fail us and cause poorer health over time. We also ignore the myriad of other factors that

> The "health" of this nation is **worse than ever,** not because people fail at weight loss but because weight-loss attempts fail us and cause poorer health over time.

influence true health—mental health, sleep, food security, joyful movement, access to non-stigmatizing healthcare, and more. Our amazing bodies will naturally change over the course of our lives. But, sadly, we keep prescribing diets in the name of "health" while ignoring the truth that body diversity and change are divine.

THE WORLD SAYS . . .

You owe everyone a number on the scale.

THE WORD SAYS . . .

If only my anguish could be weighed
and all my misery be placed on the scales!

Job 6:2

STEPPING INTO TRUTH

I pray you feel a weight lifted. We owe no one
a certain number on the scale, even when
this world tries so hard to tell us otherwise.
Spend a moment to check in with yourself.

- Where have you felt expectations around
  weight? What kind of impact does knowing these
  expectations don't come from our gracious God
  have on you?

- Sometimes we feel tremendous grief in regard
  to our past experiences around dieting and
  weight. Take some time to jot down some
  thoughts about giving up the notion that you owe
  someone a number on a scale. How might it help
  you? How might it help others? Is it possible you
  can help others see this truth?

- In Job 6:2, Job pleads to have his misery weighed
  on a scale. I think of the story of Job and the
  immense pain and loss he endured. I can't help
  but see this connection in current times. How has
  our culture's obsession with weight brought pain
  to you or someone you know?

- Isn't it amazing to know we don't owe a weight to
  anyone? To me, it's even more amazing to know
  that God never asks us to chase a number on a
  scale.

Truth #6

Seeing Diet Culture Builds Resilience

> The greatest trick the devil ever pulled was convincing Christians that oppression is godly.
>
> **Beth Allison Barr, *The Making of Biblical Womanhood***

From time to time, clients I've supported along their journeys reach out to share the various ways they see diet culture affect their lives. They're often excited to be able to see it so clearly and steer clear. Sometimes they're sad because they can see its oppression everywhere, and it feels so big and overwhelming. Other times they're angry because people in their circles fail to see it. Most messages I get these days are about how this thief shows up in places of worship—places where all bodies should be safe—which is what happened to Alex and her friends.

Alex spent her adolescent years battling an eating disorder triggered in a middle school health class. When she graduated from high school, she skipped the celebrations and went straight to treatment for her eating disorder. She worked hard to trust her recovery, and recognizing the lies of diet culture helped her do it. The lies filled her with anger and yet fueled her drive to stay well. When she returned home to her family, her confidence about feeding herself started to fade. Her family was immersed in chronic dieting and disordered eating patterns. They thought everything was "all better" because Alex had gotten treatment, so now they could go back to their typical food- and body-shaming ways.

Safe environments free of negative food, body, or diet talk are crucial for recovery. But those kinds of places are hard to find, even in homes filled with loving people. Unfortunately, even when someone does the work to see diet culture, most of us live in the waters of this culture. It is arduous and often lonely work to resist, grow in awareness, and help others see the truth.

Whether you've been a dieter or have suffered from an eating disorder, you can feel like a fish swimming upstream once you've acquired the lens that helps you see diet culture more clearly. When you're stuck in the diet cycle, you're swimming along with all the other fish. Diet culture teaches the fish that they don't have the option to go any other way. Fish that have never been above the water don't even know they're in the sea. But once we—the fish—see diet culture and begin to feed ourselves, being surrounded again by dieting and body bashing can send us right back into treacherous waters, which is what happened to Alex.

After Alex came back home to her family, she began going to church again. Her longtime family pastor suggested she join a young adult ministry group he was leading so she could meet some new friends. All was going well until the group started talking about dating woes one evening. One of Alex's friends started talking about how she'd like to date more and wondered if the group had tips. She got some standard feedback from her peers—offers to introduce her to a friend of a friend or plans for a night out. When the pastor weighed in, the situation took a turn for the worse. He told Alex's friend that going on a diet would be a good idea.

This "tending to your appearance by dieting" message is wrong on so many levels. Without having any idea about the young woman's general health, eating habits, or mental wellness, this spiritual adviser suggested a diet. Alex bravely turned up the volume on her recovery voice and let him know he was wrong, explaining that all bodies are fearfully and wonderfully made. I mean, is it possible he forgot that biblical truth?

Alex wasn't just worried about her friend; she was worried about everyone who heard the comment and all the others receiving similar advice. Alex gave the pastor a crash course in the oppression of diet culture, eating disorders, and weight bias and the harmfulness of dieting. Sometimes even good people don't know how to be open-minded, perhaps because diet culture lies about our bodies, health, and relationships are baked into both secular and seminary teachings.

Diet culture lies about our bodies, health, and relationships are baked into both secular and seminary teachings.

The process of unlearning takes a willingness to admit being wrong, and in this case the pastor wasn't. Though he chose to continue his complicity in diet culture, Alex took the initiative to declare the truth. She could now see how diet culture had infiltrated the safest of places. And she was ready to point it out everywhere. So can you.

Seeing Helps, but It Doesn't Make Resisting Diet Culture Easy

The situation with Alex and her friends turned out okay, primarily because Alex courageously pointed out the dangers of diet culture. If she hadn't dared to correct the pastor, those comments could have had more significant consequences, similar to the way her middle school health class had triggered her eating disorder.

We can be fully capable of seeing the truth about diet culture and still want to participate. Having the ability to see diet culture doesn't mean we'll never want to diet again. We're all human. We will continue to be vulnerable to its ploys. This culture preys on our need for connection and belonging, and it tries to convince us that changing our bodies will deliver the connections we crave. We're hungry for love and acceptance, and diet culture tries to sell them to us, but we don't need to fall for these lies anymore. There is a noxious arrogance in a system that thinks it can sell what only a gracious and loving God can provide. It's a gift to have our eyes opened to the truth, but it's also important to realize that when we begin to see clearly how these lies have been woven into almost every part of our society, we can be filled with anger and grief.

Several years ago, I gave a presentation on diet culture and toxic media images. I explained that the photos were altered, that the models don't look like that in real life. They don't even follow the diet or lifestyle they're trying to sell you. During the presentation, I noticed a young girl (probably twelve or thirteen years old) who seemed very upset. Now, I've been speaking to audiences on this topic for a long time, and I've become pretty good at reading a room. *Are they with me? Do they think I'm crazy? Are they bored?* This youngster was none of those. She was on the verge of tears, and she looked as if she was afraid of me. You'd have thought I had just kicked her dog.

As I packed up after the talk, her mom walked over to thank me for giving the presentation. I was curious to know more about her daughter's reaction and asked if she was okay. Her mom said, "She thought it was all real—the pictures, the bodies, the eating next to nothing—and she's seeing for the first time how she's been lied to." This sweet child was overwhelmed with anger and grief. She was riddled with sorrow that the world could so effortlessly alter images and lie to her. She was sad that all the things those lies promised—the photoshopped bodies and faces and the glamorous lives—would never be hers because they weren't even real. They didn't even belong to the people in the photos.

The emotions that come with seeing diet culture can be difficult to cope with. In addition to grief and sadness, we can feel lonely after deciding not to conform to dieting groupthink. However, by not conforming, we can find greater strength to avoid diet culture traps—like a visit to the doctor that results in cut-and-paste recommendations that tempt us to cut calories and track food or a church group contemplating doing a diet together. By not conforming, we become better equipped to root out the diet plans and "health" gimmicks that promote weight loss and tell us we need to change our bodies.

Because we're exposed to diet culture every day, we will be tempted to return to its schemes many times. But I pray you will remember the harm it has caused in so many lives, and even in your own. If the principles of diet culture worked, we wouldn't be spending our time talking about it right now; we'd just be living our lives, trusting our innate self-regulation systems to guide us, and celebrating *all the lovely bodies* in this world. We would be free.

We can all be free. Even though seeing the truth is hard, it opens the door to a life of more. More connection. More pleasure. More authenticity. More love. More peace. More gratitude. More satisfaction. And, most likely, more yummy food. Imagine you and your neighbors seeing the lies of diet culture and deciding to opt out of it together. I want an invitation to that dinner party! There would be no diet, "bad" food, or body talk—just friends, food, and thoughtful conversations. We can do it. We can be those neighbors.

Seeing Creates Resilience

You may notice the huge numbers of people who are stuck on the diet culture hamster wheel while you continue to swim upstream. Many of us have probably been there, spinning the wheel from diets to "not a diet diets" to "healthy lifestyle" plans, and so we can have compassion for our own journey and the journeys of others—journeys that will look different for all of us.

When we stand in the grocery checkout line and see a magazine cover promoting a TV doctor's recommendations for quick weight-loss plans, we know the claims are bogus and harmful. So many celebrities and celebrity doctors today have become prophets of diet culture—not because they care about you, but because they care about the big check they get from the diet industry. They use their stardom and "credibility" to sell the product and hope we'll buy the lies they're promoting. But

Many celebrities and celebrity doctors have become prophets of diet culture—not because they care about you, but because they care about the big check they get from the diet industry.

you can feel empowered to roll your eyes at diet culture and walk away. Walking away builds resilience.

If the school sends home an assignment asking a child to keep food records, conduct calorie counts, or do self-weight checks, you will know that harm is on the horizon. Teachers are simply delivering a curriculum supplied by their governing agencies. You can send a note to the teacher letting them know these lessons can lead to harmful consequences and that your child will not participate. Disengaging from diet culture builds resilience.

You may hear a pastor talk negatively about their own body or the bodies of others, and you know what they don't yet know—that assuming something is wrong with our bodies communicates a denial that our bodies are fearfully and wonderfully made, on purpose and for a purpose. It's likely you have great respect and admiration for this pastor and want them to see this truth. You can offer feedback about the harms of body shaming and diet culture. I hope you'll get a better response than Alex did. Telling her pastor that his words were dangerous didn't wake him up, but it did make her convictions even stronger. Speaking up about diet culture in safe places builds resilience.

When a friend tells you they plan to start another diet program next Monday, you can share your own story about how you've let go of diets and have been learning how diet culture keeps us further from God, not closer to him. You may know what it feels like to start letting go of all the food and body shame. Even if you're not all the way there yet, we can work on challenging diet culture together. Being in community with those who no longer want to participate in diet culture builds resilience.

As you see the weight-loss advertisements and confront the customary weight checks in medical offices, you can know that these are not the ways to measure true health. You now know that diet culture and weight bias heavily influence health education and research. If it feels safe to you, you may even address the harmful marketing materials with your provider. You have every right to feel secure in what is intended to be a safe place. Sometimes patients forget that they are the most important member of their healthcare team. You have a voice. If you can use it to promote safer places, do it! Those of us who can speak up can help those who don't yet feel safe enough to call out diet culture harms. Knowing your consent matters builds resilience.

I have people in my life who are heavily rooted in diet culture. I know this because I've repeatedly tried to help them see the negative influence, but they're not willing to consider that it's harming them or anyone else. I've had to set boundaries around the time my family and I spend with them. It's hard, but remember how the seeds of truth get planted—little comments here and there in the safe places. It's not our job to save everyone from diet culture, but we are responsible for trying to keep our circles as safe as possible. Cultivating safe places that are free of diet culture talk builds resilience.

We are capable of living a fulfilling life without absorbing the lies of diet culture. As my daughter says, "Jesus didn't create food for us to worry about eating it." However, there will be times when this truth can be hard to believe because diet culture *will* rear its ugly head and tempt

> It's not our job to save everyone from diet culture, but we are **responsible** to keep our circles as safe as possible.

us repeatedly to return to it. Remember this: Jesus does not intend for us to be in bondage to anything that could bring harm to our divinely created bodies. He intends for us to be free.

THE WORLD SAYS . . .

Diet culture is where you need to belong.

THE WORD SAYS . . .

Those who know your name trust in you,
for you, LORD, have never forsaken those who
seek you.

Psalm 9:10

STEPPING INTO TRUTH

The ability to see diet culture for what
it is leads to freedom, yet it's a freedom
that comes with many new choices.

- In what ways are you seeing the impact of diet culture?

- Have you seen it at the grocery checkout? On television? At church? On social media? In your home? At the doctor's office? It's in all the places, even when the people in these places mean well.

- Have you experienced this transition yourself— moving from diet culture to an awareness that you are, and always have been, just the way God wants you to be? That's true even as our bodies change throughout life.

- How will you continue to see the truth about diet culture? Will you bring others into your community—into your safe circles?

- Take a moment to read Psalm 9:10. In what ways can you trust God to help you reject a culture that forsakes our souls? The more we seek the Lord, the more resilient we can become in seeing cultural lies.

You Will Not Look like the Influencer, Even If They Say So

> Spiritual trauma is someone handing you an inner critic and telling you it's the voice of God.
>
> **Hillary McBride, PhD, Twitter post, April 4, 2022, 9:01 p.m.**

Years ago, I was a news channel junkie. I'd watch the news from the time I got home from work until bedtime. I'd have it on in the background while I was cooking dinner, working on my computer, having conversations in another room, or even taking a shower. The daily bombardment of death and destruction negatively influenced my life and chiseled away at my mental health. One day, when my daughter was just an infant, my anxiety was so out of control that I was teetering on the edge of losing it.

My brain couldn't handle the nonstop reports of violence and hatred in the world. I'd wake up with nightmares and lie awake with my heart racing, trying to figure out how to protect my daughter if some violent thing were to happen at the grocery store, in church, or at school. That's when I stopped. I was done with the constant news and its influence on my life. I took a news sabbatical and resolved to put better boundaries around my media consumption when I returned.

Now I get a daily news brief in my email inbox to give me control over how the information gets to me and influences me. I can skim to keep up on current events and move on. I also get a dose of what our culture calls "news" on social media. As I open my social accounts to check in with colleague groups or friends, a new type of headline seems to be more prevalent—the influencer or celebrity life update. I've seen stories like:

"This star's beach look leaves nothing to the imagination"
"This influencer's thirty-day diet program will have you
    beach ready by May"
"This famous person's girlfriend hikes in chic leggings"
"You must see this celeb's 'stay hot after baby' routine"

First of all, none of this is actually news. More importantly, these clips are exceptionally destructive. This kind of "news" about celebrities' or influencers' bodies uses the language of belonging and love in dangerous ways. It perpetuates the cultural objectification of bodies, devalues the real contributions of human beings, and makes us feel like we'll never measure up. (By the way, it's impossible to measure up because it's all smoke and mirrors.)

Welcome to the Age of Influencers

The dictionary defines an influencer as "one who exerts influence: a person who inspires or guides the actions of others; a person who is able to generate interest in something (such as a consumer product) by posting about it on social media." They're everywhere these days. You don't have to be a celebrity anymore to have influential power.

The truth is, the potential is there for all of us to be influencers. I guess I could be considered an influencer since I say and write things that may influence people. There are some great influencers out there, but we're not talking about them. We're going straight for the scary stuff. We're going to focus on the diet and fitness influencers who, sadly, use their bodies as their business cards. These influencers, in much the same way that many popular magazines do, are selling lies.

Bodies aren't business cards, but that doesn't mean people don't use them that way. From the gym selfie selling multilevel-marketing shakes to fabulous lifestyle posts—lifestyles you could have too if you just used their product—the blatant or implied "look like me" promise is a prominent marketing strategy. Marketing doesn't need to be honest or accurate; it just needs to sell products and grow influencer platforms.

Marketing doesn't need to be honest or accurate; it just needs to sell products and grow influencer platforms.

Let's start with the highly unnecessary "what I eat in a day" posts, which are everywhere. Let me tell you, as an eating disorder dietitian, I find these to be infuriating because everyone's needs are different—and in most cases really, really different. Some influencers even calculate the daily calories on their post, demonstrating just how little they eat in a day. When a teen or even an adult looks at posts like this, they may question if they're feeding themselves "right." After all, if those people eat like that and look like that, they must be doing it right, right? Wrong!

As I scan these types of posts, I have yet to see someone who reports that they eat enough food. Many of these posts show a daily intake that would be at a starvation level for adults. Now, if you're feeding a toddler, it may be enough, but I'm not sure how many toddlers are eating pretend ham and cheese sandwiches on sliced zucchini. Some of my clients and friends have fallen victim to these posts. We do a lot of undoing in my office.

Influencers often use their bodies or physical appearance as false proof of their expert qualifications, making us think we can look just like them if we just do what they say or buy their product. The truth is that you can eat just like them, but it may be intensely disordered. You can exercise just like they say they do, but it may be excessive or involve an activity you detest. You can shop at the same trendy boutique where they buy their clothes—if you can afford it—but you won't have their body or life because you will never have their genetics (or their bank account balance).

This can get tricky when the influencer is a healthcare professional like a doctor, dietitian, or therapist. These professionals should know that eating or moving in the same way that someone else eats and moves cannot make a body double. Sadly, though, they're also out there using their bodies to sell nonsense on the socials. Medical providers may post that eating "white" foods is bad for your health. (Can someone provide evidence, please? A quick Google Scholar or PubMed search yields no results.) Dietitian influencers may suggest low-calorie eating that will harm people down the road or guarantee something no one can guarantee, such as permanent weight loss. Mental health professionals may give tips for losing weight as though weight were a behavior or weight loss a behavioral health intervention; they're not. These kinds of actions violate the code of ethics for all health professionals—registered dietitians, medical doctors, therapists, all of us—whether we say these things in our offices or on the socials.[1]

It's a shame to see health professional influencers promoting such harmful practices, but it's tragic to see a ministry influencer suggesting that a body or diet like theirs is what we should pursue. When prominent people in ministry suggest that others imitate their approach to eating or that the way they eat or worship is the reason they look the way they do, the result can wound the soul. What they're peddling is not true, even if your Jesus-loving leader said it. I see these "get healthy like I did" initiatives quite frequently. We've really missed the big picture of divine body diversity. And we've ignored that our bodies, no matter how they look or what they eat, were made good by a good God. *God, help us see how the influencer, even the Christian one, isn't immune to the schemes of diet culture.*

You Don't Have to Be on Social Media to Influence or Be Influenced

Anyone can be an influencer, and you don't even have to be on social media. Your friend next door, the person down the street, or your work colleague who may say, "If you want to know why I look like this, shoot me a text or come over for coffee and I'll fill you in." Maybe it's the neighbor you invite to dinner who makes a snide comment about what you're serving but is eager to tell you all about their new diet or lifestyle plan. It could be your friend's "before and after" body pictures on Facebook. These interactions may make you question your own eating. You've been influenced. It happens to all of us, which is why we must be aware of it.

Whether these people are humans we know or accounts on the socials, influencers can feel just as trapped as anybody else. I know this because they're also my clients. Sometimes when I get furious with these people, I have to remind myself that we all swim in the sea of diet culture.

Tam was a coach with a big following. She was terrified that she would lose her clients, social platform, and income if her body changed. All of her eggs were in one basket—her physical appearance. She suffered from disordered eating practices for years, some attributed to her sport and some learned in her home while growing up.

Her weight control behaviors grew more severe from year to year. As her body aged and changed normally, she feared losing work. She knew she was trapped and couldn't see a way out. That's when she came to see me. When Tam told me about her restrictive routines to "keep her body in check," I worried about her medical safety. She was a ticking time bomb, and no one knew it, not even her family.

Tam said she had gone to the doctor to get help a few weeks before landing in my office. The visit didn't go well. She told the doctor about her restrictive eating, extreme exercise regimen, racing heart, and dizziness. The doctor, who was not trained to assess disordered eating, looked at her and said, "You're the picture of health. Keep doing what you're doing," and sent her on her way. Tam told me she felt so bad that day that she didn't know if she would wake up the next morning. She realized at that moment that her looks had nothing to do with her health, and the pressure of using her body as her business card just might kill her.

She also realized that she wasn't hurting only herself; she was sending harmful messages to those who worked with her or followed her. She'd made the key to health look so easy, but she was telling a lie. And she resolved that if she was going to be a person with influence over others, she was going to have to be an honest one. Tam didn't want anyone else to suffer in the same way. It was time to come clean.

As she began to feed her body enough food and decrease her exercise workouts, her body changed, as most bodies do. She started sleeping better. She had the necessary mental energy to hang out with her kids. Tam also told her clients and followers that she had learned she wasn't eating enough before and was wrong. She started to focus more on sport skills with her clients than aesthetics. And she told them that any body they showed up in was a good body. Not one client left her. Tam felt good about showing up as her authentic self, without the burden of having to maintain a certain body type. While coming clean wasn't easy, she was *not* turning back to diet culture.

We Can Change Our Minds about Our Bodies and Our Influence

Our physical bodies may hold some form of social currency in this messed-up culture, but that doesn't translate to health. And it means nothing in heaven. We must get comfortable ignoring the false promises and false prophets of diet culture.

If any social media influencer makes you question your body's goodness, it's time to unfollow. If pretend news about celebrity bodies makes you feel inadequate or not good enough, block it, delete it, or scroll on. Don't be afraid to set boundaries regarding food and body talk, even if it's with your neighbor or coworker. This could be a moment of great influence and opportunity for you both. Can our homes, offices, and minds become the safe places we all need? I believe they can, provided we are willing to allow our fed and authentic selves to show up. Accepting body diversity can be hard in our culture, but it's a lot easier when we're not trying to be someone else.

THE WORLD SAYS . . .

Following the actions of an influencer
will bring health and belonging.

THE WORD SAYS . . .

Whoever loves God is known by God.

1 Corinthians 8:3

STEPPING INTO TRUTH

We've been under a spell in our culture—a spell that creates the illusion that a specific look equates to health and expertise. But it just doesn't add up.

- Has an influencer taken advantage of you? I think at some point this has happened to all of us. Whether it's the supplement-pushing buddy in your Bible study group, a neighbor pressuring you to join WW or Noom, or the verse-spouting, diet-selling supermom on social media, the pressure is on to join a community that has learned to use the language of belonging. You don't belong there. You belong to the kingdom of God.

- In what ways have you seen the influence of the influencer show up in your life? Was it on social media? Did it come from someone close to you? Was it a health professional or ministry leader?

- Knowing what you know now, how can you protect yourself from false promises and prophets?

- Have you ever been an influencer? What would you do in the same way or differently now?

- Take a moment to read and think about 1 Corinthians 8:3. We're often searching for belonging in this world. But we are already known and loved. We don't have to influence or be influenced to receive it.

Truth # 8

You Can Detox from Social Media and Trackers

Social media is really not equipped for the complexity of humans and their feelings.

Matt Haig, author of *Reasons to Stay Alive*

Part of my job involves supervising other dietitians and health professionals. I have the honor of helping others work through tough cases, guiding them to navigate differences in opinion between treatment teams, and supporting their work with clients and their families. A session doesn't go by that we don't talk about how social media, specific apps, and trackers can prevent clients from healing. Diet culture has us outsourcing our inner wisdom to influencers, artificial intelligence, and fancy calculators.

We've become dependent on external guidance in various aspects of our lives. Of course, certain external guides are extremely helpful—checking the weather forecast to know how to dress for the day or using a maps app to help us navigate the best routes, for example. The pandemic made grocery selection and delivery via an app superconvenient. Many of today's options offer great benefits. But in the context of diet culture, there's a strong possibility that some apps and trackers will have a profoundly negative impact.

In the last several years, social media and trackers have played a significant role in the suffering of my clients. Although some health and fitness professionals recommend using these tools, and many of my friends use them, I regularly see them cause more harm than good. Often they become another idol, just like the scale. *Did I check to see what that influencer posted today? I forgot to post my workout. I wasn't able to track my breakfast macros on time. Darn, I didn't get my activity counted for today.* We'll outsource our God-given wisdom to these apps and trackers if we're not careful. Constant social media use and obsessive tracking can also steal our time with God. Not everything made for good is used for good—particularly in the hands of diet culture.

A Social Media "Detox"

Alicia deleted all of her social media accounts once she realized the devastating toll they were taking on her mind and body. The daily bombardment of pseudo-health and diet posts led to struggles with orthorexia—an unhealthy fixation on being healthy. Her new "health" habits prevented her from traveling for work and eating out with her friends. Every day became a grueling process of reading labels, rereading labels, and making every meal from scratch. Alicia was exhausted, and so was everyone around her. She was ready for a social media detox.

As we got to know each other, Alicia told me about some of the accounts she'd been following that were causing her distress. At first, she thought she was just getting "healthy" eating and exercise tips. As her mental and physical health deteriorated, she realized that those posts had only encouraged the development of her eating disorder. She knew she had to be done with it, at least for a while.

Even when you think you have the tightest controls on your accounts and do your best to limit your time on social media, you don't control what you see; the ever-changing algorithms do. You are not entirely in charge of what you consume on social media unless you choose not to consume it at all. It's the only detox out there I can get behind.

Wait, but You're on the Socials

I use social media too. That's how I've met many of you! There is certainly some value in it. I follow great accounts that bring me beautiful blessings, expose me to life truths, and make me think. I like to post hiking pictures for my friends and family to see and thoughts about diet culture in "safe" places for my followers. It's where many of us spend time and connect. We just need to be vigilant if we continue in that space because the socials don't care about us or our well-being. Ultimately, they only care about what we are willing to buy.

As more evidence of harm emerges, I have become aware that I'm responsible for setting my own boundaries when it comes to social media consumption. While I use it mainly for my business, I try to limit my time and curate a feed of accounts that are helpful to me. That doesn't mean I don't see awful and triggering stuff (I'm not immune to it). I do a lot of reporting, unfollowing, and blocking, particularly on Facebook and Instagram. I just reported an account containing "before and after" pictures that promoted a diet product with a lot of disordered eating suggestions. We must set our own boundaries around social media consumption.

Platforms that are more appearance-focused, such as Instagram and TikTok, tend to be the most dangerous. Research suggests that viewing body-based posts can lead to body image disturbances, particularly in young women.[1] Reading appearance-related comments (such as "You look great!" or "Nice legs!") on Instagram can increase the viewer's body dissatisfaction as well.[2] Another study across many social media platforms revealed a dose-related response: the more time someone spends using and viewing social media, the greater the likelihood this person will suffer from disordered eating behaviors or eating concerns.[3]

The evidence is startling, and we must guard our minds and hearts from what I believe to be one of the enemy's favorite tools—social media. If we're constantly on our phones, comparing the way we eat, move, and look with the way others do, that doesn't leave much room to celebrate having our own fearfully and wonderfully

> A culture fixated on female thinness is not an **obsession** about female beauty, but an obsession about female **obedience**. Dieting is the most potent political sedative in women's history; a quietly mad population is a tractable one.
>
> Naomi Wolf, *The Beauty Myth*

made bodies. Don't forget that these photos are almost always edited or filtered (lies, all lies). There's a reason some people use the hashtag #unfiltered—nearly every picture out there *is* filtered or manipulated somehow. It's time to draw some boundary lines. Let's start deleting and blocking.

As you start deleting accounts that make you question your body or tempt you to restrict your nutrition, think about other external controls or triggers you'll need to evaluate. For many of my clients like Alicia, this means they start deleting apps and disabling certain functions on their smartwatches. Grabbing an umbrella when your app or smartwatch suggests that rain is coming is great; skipping lunch because MyFitnessPal says you've already eaten too many calories isn't.

"My Watch Says I Don't Need That Much"

I can't tell you how many times I've heard my clients say, "My watch says I don't need that much." My clients are often very confident in the smartwatch calculations of their body's needs. Why wouldn't they be? We've been taught that our devices are smarter than we are at controlling our bodies. Hear me very clearly: *that is not true.* No tracker or wearable can replace interoceptive awareness, measure continuous hormone shifts, or detect your stress levels. Those are inside jobs that your body was divinely created to do.

When we add to our devices apps that track our calories, food, or workouts, we'll often get push notifications based on a default setting. That default tends to be starvation-like levels of calories (don't forget just how off base those are).

Fitness trackers may tell us to push harder or put in more steps. They may let us know that we've "earned" food (which isn't a thing, since the body needs food, period). Many of these apps

WHAT IS INTEROCEPTIVE AWARENESS?

Interoceptive awareness is the ability to sense what is happening in your body in the present moment. You may feel your heart rate increase when you send a final project to your boss or a gentle emptiness in your stomach when you're ready for an afternoon snack. The ability to notice these sensations is interoceptive awareness, which is an integral aspect of mental and physical wellness—an aspect that diet culture conflicts with and often silences. When you lose your interoceptive awareness ability, finding it again can take a very long time.

---

combine food intake tracking and fitness logging with additional wearables. When we're tracking an already low intake and our fitness calculations suggest we only get a few more calories for our exercise, disordered eating is lurking just a small step away.

I know I'm frequently using the terms "disordered eating" and "disordered behaviors" in this book. And if I failed to make it clear in part 1, I want to make it *crystal* clear now. Dieting or restricting our caloric intake and obsessively tracking our calories and movement are disordered behaviors, whether a doctor or dietitian recommended these practices or not. They *are* disordered. If you're still stuck in these habits, don't beat yourself up. Diet culture sets us up to be sucked in. I promise you're not alone.

Alicia didn't realize the negative impact of these practices until the tracking and social scrolling she had been doing left her with debilitating anxiety around her food and movement. One day, we talked about getting rid of her trackers (remember, she had already ditched social media). She had a lot of trouble trusting me that she needed far more energy (or calories) than her smartwatch was calculating. She was in complete disbelief actually. That's because not enough is almost always the default mode of trackers.

Her skepticism wasn't new to me. I am no stranger to talking people off the ledge of diet culture. So we dove right into the evidence. Alicia, a healthcare professional herself, read over a few articles we'd talked about in session. The first paper she reviewed was about using MyFitnessPal for calorie tracking and whether or not it contributed to the development of the participants' eating disorders. The female participants in this study had recently been discharged from treatment for their eating disorders. Almost 75 percent of those in the study reported using MyFitnessPal, and of those, more than 80 percent said it contributed to their eating disorder.[4] Another study found similar results regarding men using MyFitnessPal and its role in their eating disorder symptoms.[5]

Alicia decided she needed to disable the fitness and calorie tracking information being pushed to her smartwatch and delete the apps contributing to her symptoms. We started working on getting her back in touch with her own body's wisdom, and she began to practice sensing her own needs instead of allowing a device to guide her. It was hard at first, but she regained trust in her divine vessel and made a full recovery. Detoxing from harmful social accounts and apps can be challenging, but remembering who made you and trusting your good body is a

> Dieting or restricting our caloric intake and obsessively tracking our calories and movement are **disordered behaviors,** whether the doctor or dietitian recommended these practices or not.

freedom I want for everyone. It requires patience and diligence because it will probably take longer than you think, but it is so worth it.

Are All Wearables and Smart Devices Bad?

Not all wearables and smart devices are bad, but intention matters. If you're using the device to shrink your body or count calories, you're serving diet culture, not your health. Some people like to monitor their heart rate during exercise, and others may use a wearable for sleep. These are intentions that can help with performance or increase awareness of factors that may influence health. Are smart devices necessary? No. Can they be useful sometimes? Yes. My husband tracks our GPS on his watch when we're hiking, and I map our route on my phone. This is useful to us because we don't want to get lost. It has nothing to do with calories burned.

I'm "connected" enough at this point in my life, so I've decided I don't want a smartwatch, even though to get texts on my wrist seems really cool. That part is tempting to me, but I know I'd be more distracted than I already am, and I just may be tempted by some of those default numbers. The bottom line is that none of us are immune. We get to decide as individuals how to set boundaries around social media, smart devices, and apps in order to keep our brains in check, our bodies fed, and our hearts pointed to God.

THE WORLD SAYS . . .
This app knows what you need better
than you do—and better than God does.
Just follow me and my calculations.

THE WORD SAYS . . .

You have searched me, LORD,
and you know me.
You know when I sit and when I rise;
you perceive my thoughts from afar.
You discern my going out and my lying down;
you are familiar with all my ways.

Psalm 139:1–3

STEPPING INTO TRUTH

We live in a very interesting time. Social media instantly alerts us to disasters while our watches beep at us to get up and move. Sometimes it feels great to be in the know, and sometimes our beeping wrists can start a shame spiral. In this sneaky culture, we can forget that we control what we let in and allow to influence us. A perfect God gave you what you need—your unique design and the ability to listen to your own body. And our great God *knows* you.

- Let's start with social media. Do you follow certain accounts that make you question the way you eat, move, dress, or care for yourself? If so, make a quick list of them.

- Do these accounts trigger a desire to engage in diet culture? If so, are you willing to delete or unfollow these accounts? If yes, great. Take that, diet culture! If not, spend a few moments reflecting on what is standing in the way and causing your hesitation.

- Now let's talk about wearables and smartwatches. Do you have these items? What is the true intention? Do you want to begin to create boundaries with regard to your use of these tools?

- Read Psalm 139:1–3. We may use apps and gadgets in our lives, but do they truly *know* us? Think about how much our great God knows us and how, if we reconnect with ourselves, we can know and trust our bodies without external controls.

You Are You on Purpose

There's nothing wrong with having aspirations or doing your best. But having an expectation of perfection turns life into a performance, and it comes at a big price. You lose your authenticity and connection to your true self.

Evelyn Tribole, *Intuitive Eating for Every Day*

When I was in junior high, I spent time in the summer with my grandmother and her sisters in the mountains of North Carolina. We'd go for walks, play games, take pictures (with film!), cook family recipes, and take scenic drives on the Blue Ridge Parkway. I loved the time with Nanny and her sisters in that little mountain village.

Each morning, Nanny and her sisters drank coffee on the back deck overlooking those beautiful mountains. We sat on big wooden chairs and watched the sun fade away each evening. Just as the sun dipped beyond the horizon, flying squirrels came out from the trees and visited us. (I have actual photo evidence.)

On the days when it rained, we sat and listened to raindrops hitting every single green thing around the cabin.

Nanny and her sisters decorated the cabin for Christmas, even though we were there in the middle of the summer. They each had families of their own and didn't see each other during the holidays. So Christmas in July it was! I had so much fun helping Nanny wrap gifts and get ready for time in the mountains. What fierce love they had for each other and me! I'm so fond of those memories.

One day, we were out walking. I distinctly remember walking ahead of everyone—it was impossible for me to slow down in those days. While the sisters were chatting behind me, I heard one of them say, "She's got those Salyer calves." Being a junior high kid, I wasn't sure what to make of that comment. Did that mean my calves were good? Did that mean something was wrong with them? I mean, after all, wasn't I a Salyer too?

I thought about that comment off and on as I sprinted in the 200-meter race, jumped hurdles as fast as I could, and tumbled through my gymnastics career. As I got older and heard more diet and body talk from pretty much everyone I encountered, including Nanny and her sisters, I realized the comment wasn't a compliment. It meant my calves were too big, too strong, and just not what the women in the family found desirable. How could something be wrong with those calves? They had done so many good things for me!

These "Salyer calves" have given me the very fortunate experience of being able-bodied. They have carried me to the other side of this world for mission work. They hold me up while I speak on platforms across the nation about rooting out the lies of diet culture. They haul my body up and over the mountains I hike out west. Nanny and her sisters learned that something was wrong with their power somewhere along the way. They

FAMILIAL SEEDS OF DOUBT

Our conversations matter. Even when we don't think little ears are paying attention, they hear everything. Even when we speak with good intentions, seeds of doubt can be planted in young minds. Here are a few examples of comments made by adult family members and the various ways these comments tend to land on a young one's heart. You may have heard similar words growing up.

Seeds of Doubt	Plant False Belief
Did you notice that Aunt Linda has gained weight?	Body change is something to be feared. Weight changes are always bad.
Dad, do you really need a second helping?	Bodies cannot be trusted. Food cannot be trusted.
Mom, you have diabetes. Are you supposed to be eating that muffin?	It's okay to micromanage or judge others' bodies or decisions. People with diabetes can't eat muffins and similar kinds of foods.
Heart disease runs in our family, Jack. We need to be very careful about what we eat.	Strictly controlling food selections will keep you free from disease (and living in fear).
Why did you eat so much of that, Sarah? It's so bad for you.	Something must be wrong with me for liking certain foods. I am a bad kid. I can't trust myself.
I can't believe I ate so much yesterday. I'd better eat less and work out extra hard today.	Food must be earned. Eating more than I usually do requires restriction or compensation.

had concluded that they needed to change their bodies. And let me tell you, I heard about Nanny's body dissatisfaction until she died.

I know deep down that if Nanny and her sisters had known how diet culture was hurting them and those around them, they never would have spoken negatively about bodies. I know that if they had seen how diet culture pushed them to judge themselves and others, they would have stopped. I know they'd be proud of those Salyer calves now, but mostly of the person they hold up today. But even if they weren't, I'm reminded that *I am fearfully and wonderfully made*. And so are you!

As I look back at that particular Christmas in July at the cabin in the mountains, I know that body hatred is not a gift I have to receive. Whether we like it or not, our family of origin is our heritage. Not all of us have wonderful or affectionate memories of our earthly families, but we do have a firm foundation in a loving heavenly Father. And our God doesn't make junk. Nanny didn't have the chance to see diet culture for what it is and understand how it interfered with her life. But we do.

Look Around at This Beautiful Collection of Humans

We are different on purpose. You know what I'm going to say next—I know you do. Body diversity is divine. Our bodies are spectacular because they are inextricably tied to our hearts and souls. Think about it. The Holy Spirit is embodied within us. There isn't an unworthy body out there. No matter your skin color, level of ability, body size, gender, bank account balance, or language, you are you because a great God made you that way. There is no body hierarchy in the kingdom of God. That is the gospel truth.

Sadly, this isn't always the world's truth. The body hierarchy of this world tries very hard to control us and sometimes succeeds at telling us a different story. But we must not allow this world to deny the fact that we're all image bearers. We have to claim this truth for ourselves, no matter how this world may tell lies. And if we have bodies that fall in a more "acceptable" place in this world's body hierarchy, we can use this standing, this privilege, to make this world a safer place for all bodies. We have an obligation to God and to our neighbors to do so.

> God saves you *in* your body, not *from* your body.
>
> Nadia Bolz-Weber, "Human Bodies and the Image of God," a sermon on shame and healing

We Do Not Need to Conform

We can experience belonging without diminishing or restricting our authentic selves. If we want to give the gift of our authentic selves to others and help them do the same, we must reject all attempts to measure up to unrealistic ideals.

God knew us before we were born. Just like a fingerprint, we are unique on purpose. Each of us is an extraordinary miracle—including those who look or think differently than we do. If we accept this truth for ourselves, we must also accept this truth for others.

It's also true that these miraculous bodies change over time, even though diet culture denies it. We've seemingly made it out of the worst surges of the worldwide pandemic that spanned the globe. I've seen countless posts and articles that find fault with waistlines and body changes during and after the pandemic. It baffles me how we overlook the miracle that these bodies can expand, survive, and endure such trauma!

At the time of my writing, the world has lost nearly 6.7 million people due to COVID-19.[1] Any one of us could have been included in that statistic. Meanwhile, I've seen ministry leaders comment on their bodies with disdain because they've gone up a size in their jeans, ignoring the fact that they made it through the pandemic. We are built for change. A great God made our bodies adaptable and resilient. That is the sermon I

We are built for **change.** A great God made our bodies adaptable and resilient.

want all of us to hear. That's the ministry influencer's post I want to read. You resilient, adaptable, miraculous creation of a human, you—you are here! Your body is good. Get some new jeans that fit your amazing here-and-now body and move on with your miraculous self. And go tell your neighbor they're amazing and to go and do the same. That's the sermon I want to hear!

We Don't Need to Be Shiny and New

We can't reinvent or make better something that God has already created good. Does that mean there's nothing we can do to our bodies or our appearance? Absolutely not. You may want to dress up and wear fun clothes. You may want to wear shimmery eye shadow and fun nail polish. You may want to have pink hair, which is my daughter's preferred summer color. You may love getting your hair done with a fun new style. You may want to lift weights to feel strong. You may want to run a race or hike a tough trail to feel challenged. Celebrating your body in these ways is fine, as long as celebrating your body is what you're truly doing.

It's *why* we do these things that matters. Is your intention to celebrate yourself and your autonomy? Or do you feel you have to conform to this world? Whatever you do, do it for you, the one and only divinely made you—not anyone else. And surround yourself with people who are willing to do the same.

Sometimes my daughter hangs out with me in my bathroom while I'm getting ready for work or church. I've never been particularly good at putting on makeup and styling my hair, but occasionally I like to try. One day as I was getting ready for work, my daughter asked me why I was putting on makeup. I thought about how my answer would land on her heart before responding. I told her I knew I didn't need to wear makeup and that no one needs to, but sometimes I like to sparkle just for myself. It was the answer that day and has been the answer many times thereafter. And from time to time, I check myself to make sure that's still my motivation. But even on days when it feels a little harder to believe (I live in this hard place too), I pray it will always be true for her.

> yeah, she fell.
> she got distracted
> lost her direction
> made some mistakes
> broke some promises
> forgot who she was . . .
> but she got up.
>
> Nakeia Homer, well-being educator and author of *I Hope This Helps*

If it's not true for you now, I pray it will be someday. You are the you God intended you to be. I am the me God intended me to be—"Salyer calves" and all, those calves that have carried me through so much. You are you because God wanted you.

THE WORLD SAYS . . .

Just be like and look like everyone else.

THE WORD SAYS . . .

I praise you because I am fearfully and
wonderfully made;
your works are wonderful,
I know that full well.

Psalm 139:14

STEPPING INTO TRUTH

As I've gotten older, I've become much better at feeling at home with myself. It hasn't always been easy. You may have experienced things as you grew up that made you question your authentic self. It's not the fault of our families. Diet culture is the tool of the enemy. Seeds of doubt can be planted early in our lives, which can lead to hiding, pretending, conforming, and even harmful behaviors. You're not alone.

- Is your story like mine—a story in which seeds of doubt about your body were planted early in your life?

- Do you have a story that impacted the way you show up in the world—as the real you or the conforming you? I pray you feel safe to love, care for, and express the real you.

- Have you planted seeds of doubt in the hearts of others you know and influence? I think we all have, and it's never too late to be honest about a change of heart. Grace will get us through.

- Read Psalm 139:14. Write down the words of this verse and weave your name into it. Read it aloud. Read it again. You are you on purpose—so that you will know you are fearfully and wonderfully made.

Truth #10

You Can Choose Your Legacy

> When I stand before God at the end of my life, I would hope that I would not have a single bit of talent left, and could say, "I used everything you gave me."
>
> **Erma Bombeck**

I love getting updates from former clients. The updates usually come in the form of emails. I'll see a name from the past and click on the message, eager to see what's new with them. The messages often start with a report on a surreal job opportunity or an exciting life event. Even though they no longer sit across from me in my office, I still have the great honor of learning from them as their lives have moved on.

As they share their experiences, they invariably circle around to their gratitude for having discovered the truth about diet culture and the ways this revelation has helped set them free. They're at a point in their lives they couldn't have imagined when they were wrapped up in a destructive relationship with food, their body, and diet culture. This freedom has given them the energy and mental space to live in a way they didn't know was possible.

When we can't see the truth about diet culture, it's like looking through a distorted lens that doesn't show the complete picture—the way a camera lens fails to capture a peripheral view. When we can see diet culture and reject its allure, life can be like experiencing a beautiful place you've only dreamed of or appreciating in person artwork that you'd only seen in photos. It's like seeing the ocean for the first time—both overwhelmingly powerful and breathtakingly beautiful.

I remember the first time I saw Michelangelo's *David*. I had only seen pictures in tourist books of this giant-killer carved out of marble. Nothing had prepared me for seeing the sculpture with my very own eyes. I wasn't much of an art lover early in my life. In my mind, renowned art pieces were just items tourists could check off a list. But when I saw *David*, everything I thought about art changed.

The more than five-hundred-year-old marble *David* resides safely within the walls of the Gallery of the Academy of Florence. When I rounded the corner with all the other tourists who had come to see *David*, it took my breath away. I stopped in my tracks, so taken aback by my own reaction. He was literally larger than life, standing seventeen feet tall and sparkling from the light shining in from the windows. Tears filled my eyes because he was more magnificent than I could have imagined.

Ever since this experience, the fight between David and Goliath has become more to me than a famed Bible story. It is a metaphor for the battle between good and evil. It is a reminder that a small, swordless human being can defeat even the largest and most cunning of giants when armed with the truth.

You and I are the Davids of this world. Diet culture is our Goliath. And seeing this truth is our victory. This is what my clients are attesting to in their emails—that seeing the truth has set them free. Seeing the truth has offered them something they didn't think was possible.

> You and I are the **Davids** of this world. Diet culture is our **Goliath.**

So Much Is Waiting for You on the Other Side

When you're no longer entrenched in diet culture, you can live well without feeling controlled by the numbers. You can be free to trust your divine design.
And you can find what was lost when you feed yourself. You may find lost relationships. You may find lost hobbies. You may find lost dreams and callings. You may find the bravery you thought had vanished. You may find the strength to fight for what you believe. You may even find the courage to walk away from whatever makes you feel like you need to shrink or be silent. You are a force of nature. You are an image bearer with a purpose. It's time to walk away from the thief and into your life.

Will you reconnect with yourself? Will you reconnect with others? Will you help others to see, heal, and break free? Your legacy can be different when your headspace is no longer held hostage by diet culture's lies and obsession with numbers.

As you feed yourself, perhaps you'll find yourself feeding others as well. You will feed them the truth. You will feed them food you've reclaimed from your culture and your good memories. In healing yourself, you have the potential to heal those in your circle of influence—a parent, sibling, cousin, friend, partner, child. Or it may be a teacher or pastor or your doctor or social followers.

Seeing someone close to you live well, in whatever body God has gifted them, outside the walls of diet culture demonstrates that it can be done. That doesn't mean it will always be easy. I don't think the enemy stops firing his flaming arrows this side of heaven. But it does mean that you now know you need a shield and you know when to use it.

Our Legacy Will Not Change in Silence

If we don't want to pass on a legacy steeped in diet culture, we must call out untruths before they can take root. Sometimes our shields will look like boundaries. Just the other day, a friend of mine was talking about how her kids had overheard her adult friends talking about the way they restrict their eating in hopes of changing their bodies. My friend and I talked through this scenario because she was worried about her kids and what would happen to them when she wouldn't be there to shield them from the flaming arrows.

She had told her friends that she didn't believe in dieting and that all bodies are good bodies that deserve adequate and consistent nourishment. She also added, "Please don't talk negatively about food or bodies around my children. Those words can hurt them for a lifetime." Setting this boundary was hard for her, but she knew that letting the lies of diet culture plant seeds in her kids' hearts would be far worse.

Boundaries yield resilience, and resilience can keep the seeds of untruth from settling in. Having conversations about the lies of diet culture and setting caring boundaries is like activating a force field of protection. One day, when her kids are off on their own and experience the deceits of diet culture, they'll be more likely to recognize that those words and practices are lies.

Boundaries must be set everywhere. We can and must speak truth and protection from harm in all the places—in our homes, schools, churches, medical offices, and workplaces. You may decide to talk to your boss about the toxic conversations going on in your workplace around food and bodies. It may be time to leave a comment card at church. You may want to meet with your pastor to talk about the "Jesus is the bread of life, but you shouldn't eat bread" comments in the sermon. You may decide to ask your doctor to take down the diet culture posters in their office. When the good food, bad food, and body weight–based assignments come home from school, it may be time to teach your children that they can opt out of diet culture lessons.

Having conversations about the lies of diet culture and setting caring boundaries is like activating a force field of protection.

Not only can you use your shield, but you can also be the shield. We must be the shield because not everyone can see diet culture all around them. I didn't see it for years, even as a health professional. It's not someone's fault they can't see it. That's what diet culture wants. But once you do see it, you can't unsee it, and I believe if you made it this far in this book, you don't want to perpetuate it either. Diet culture is the Goliath around every turn. Remember, you are David armed with the truth, and you can help those around you see!

Not everyone is willing to open their eyes and see. Some people are so entrenched and invested in diet culture and its prejudicial body hierarchy that no amount of evidence or seeing you live freely will convince them to disengage. While you may want

> The hardest thing about implementing **boundaries** is accepting that some people won't like, understand, or agree with yours. Once you grow beyond pleasing others, setting your standards becomes easier. Not being liked by everyone is a small consequence when you consider the overall reward of healthier relationships.
>
> Nedra Glover Tawwab,
> *Set Boundaries, Find Peace*

to help everyone escape the grasp of diet culture (and believe me, I do), it is not your job to change the hearts and minds of everyone. You can plant a seed of truth, but you're not responsible for making it grow. You must protect your heart, mind, and energy with your own boundaries, because if you don't, getting sucked back in is a real possibility.

They'll Say You've Let Yourself Go

Walking away from the false beliefs of diet culture and into a full life can be challenging for some to understand. If you're on the receiving end of someone's defensive food and body rules, these judgments can feel downright mean. You may hear things like, "How can you just let yourself go?" Those comments aren't about you; they expose the fear of those who speak them. The comments about letting yourself go come from our programmed belief that we must conform to the ways of this world to be healthy or worthy.

I want you to know that letting yourself go is a beautiful thing. In fact, letting ourselves go may be just what we need to uncover the path to a new legacy—a legacy defined by the celebration of the bodies God gave us.

Let's start by letting go of the feeling that we need to be silent. We will let go of the cultural desire to be small. I pray that all of us will find our voices and take up every bit of space we need in this world. We can let go of the cultural expectation to be at war with our bodies. Letting ourselves go results in a wholehearted acceptance of being fearfully and wonderfully made, even on the hard days. We will let go of questioning that truth because *nothing* can separate us from the love of God.

Go ahead, let go of the lie that diet culture will lead us to health. Letting yourself go means that you and a loving God decide what "health" this side of heaven will look like for you. Letting yourself go means no acronym like "BMI" can determine your health or define your righteousness. Letting go means you know full well that no diet plan or promise of body change wrapped in a Bible verse will get you closer to God, for God is already with you. Let yourself go to find nourishment and health in the ways you see fit. Move on without the lies of diet culture and its false prophets.

And praise the Lord that letting yourself go means the idols of diet culture can no longer hold you hostage. They can no longer hold you in their grip of despair once you've decided to break free. Go for a walk in nature because it fills your soul and calms your mind, not because you have steps to count. Let go of the worldly currency of weight, calories, and sizes. Goodbye, pretend metrics of worth and goodness. We are letting you go! Before the numbers and the diets, we were loved, and after the numbers, we will still be loved, for we have *always* been loved and *always* been enough.

Letting go means your eyes are wide open. Letting go means you can help others see as well. When those who can't yet see continue to say, "You're letting yourself go," you can agree. That's exactly what you're doing—letting go of worldly ideals and judgments. Maybe one day they'll join you. I pray they will—because you are letting yourself go to live a fed, full, purpose-filled life.

You're letting yourself go to love, accept, and appreciate who you are because it's the surest route to also love your neighbor. You're letting go of the expectations. You're letting go of planting doubt in the minds and hearts of children that make them think their bodies aren't good. You're letting go of questioning whether what you eat is just right or too much. You're letting go of the false requirement to participate in diet culture. Letting go means never second-guessing the desire to feed yourself.

They will say we are letting ourselves go. Let them say it. What a magnificent gift it is to let go of body distrust! It's time to pull up the weeds of doubt for good and let it all go. We will break these chains and let go of diet culture's strongholds together. And it will be glorious.

THE WORLD SAYS . . .

You cannot overcome the giant of diet culture without "letting yourself go."

THE WORD SAYS . . .

Stand firm then, with the belt of truth buckled around your waist, with the breastplate of righteousness in place, and with your feet fitted with the readiness that comes from the gospel of peace. In addition to all this, take up the shield of faith, with which you can extinguish all the flaming arrows of the evil one.

Ephesians 6:14–16

STEPPING INTO TRUTH

Here we are at the end. We are moving along in the journey of rejecting a pervasive cultural force so we can feed ourselves and step into our divine design together. What an incredible and challenging journey this unlearning and relearning can be!

- Weeds we thought were fully eradicated still sprout up from time to time. What weeds have you had to pull up over and over?

- Could these weeds be tied to an inheritance and legacy you're now ready to reject?

- What steps can you take to keep the weeds from reemerging?

- How can you help pull the weeds of doubt now that you know you don't have to conform to diet culture? The unlearning and relearning don't end. We can let go of our need to always get it right.

- What else will you let go of? Will you challenge others to let go with you?

- Are there boundaries you can set to protect yourself and those in your circle of influence?

- Take a moment to read Ephesians 6:14–16. Beloved, the flaming arrows may not come to an end in our lifetimes, but we have a good God who gave us good and diverse bodies. Pick up your shield of faith and step into a fed and free life.

I pray you'll pick up this book whenever you need encouragement. I pray you will have a community of people who will band together to expose the lies and live the truth. Those of us who go against the grain need to deliberately plant the seeds that can bring others to the truth of our divine design. I pray that the tide will turn one day and that diet culture will become the exception, not the rule. And when it does, we will be there to welcome our fellow image bearers to the shore. And I pray that you will never forget to feed yourself.

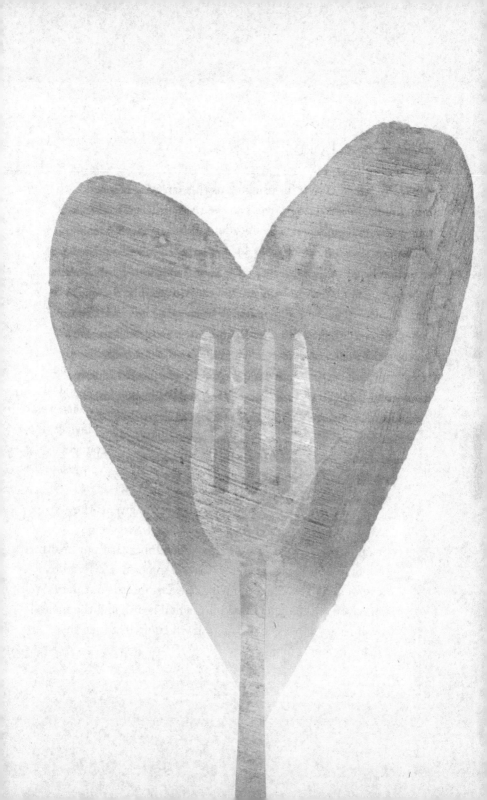

Dear Lord,

Thank you for bringing us this far. We are filled with gratitude that our eyes can see the stumbling blocks that impede our journey—for diet culture has created such a perilous path. We pray for clarity so that we can honor and nourish these diverse bodies that are fearfully and wonderfully made by you. Lord, help us remember this is true for our neighbors as well. Help us keep all bodies safe.

Heavenly Father, remind us in the midst of medical appointments that we mean so much to you, no matter what a scale says or doesn't say. Give us strength to stand against harms that may come our way, even in the safest of places. Help us see that it's the enemy at work. Give us eyes to see when it's time to disconnect from harmful devices, influencers, and social media. Lord, we want to connect with you and your kingdom. We must look up. We must reconnect with our neighbors face-to-face.

If we choose to pursue earthly health, give us the knowledge and peaceful awareness that there are no guarantees. O dear Lord, help us remember that our health is not a moral obligation, for it is not something offered to everyone in this life, but loving our neighbors is our duty. We pray you will help us value our mental health and the mental wellness of others, and that you will equip us to see the many helpers among us.

We long to be at the celebration feast with you, Jesus. Remind us that we need nourishment for daily living, and that feeding ourselves is required for a life of purpose— for you have given us the blessing of all foods. And, dearest Lord, we are so very grateful you've made this beautiful palette of human beings, each unique in ways only you could have designed. Guide us, Lord, in a spirit of togetherness, to call out and rebuke diet culture, because we will no longer allow it to be our legacy.

Amen.

Acknowledgments

This book has been on my heart and mind for nearly a decade. Those closest to me have wrestled with truth and untruths right along with me, and I am so grateful. My daughter, C. C., just may be my number one fan and diet culture fighter. Thank you, sweet girl. Brian, thank you for supporting me in this journey, even when it felt like a dead end at times. I love you both so much. I also want to thank my parents, sister, and in-laws for their unwavering belief in me.

There are so many people who have loved and supported me. I'm honored to acknowledge them with my deepest gratitude. Thank you to:

- Every single one of my clients, current and past—you trusted me to support your journey, but you taught me so much more. Thank you from the bottom of my heart.
- My Memphis supervision group—you know who you are, sweet friends. You took a baby dietitian under your wings and facilitated my growth as a person and a clinician.
- Mary Ann Ruff—you stood behind this message, supported me, and prayed for me from the moment I shared my vision with you.

- Evelyn Tribole, MS, RDN, CEDS-S, for saying, "Don't wait to get your book out into the world."
- Greta Jarvis, MS, for your help on the socials, podcasts, and editing.
- Wendy Jo Peterson, MS, RDN, and Rebecca Scritchfield, RDN, for years of friendship and guidance and for being my professional soulmates.
- Shelley Boyd for your friendship, walks, and editing skills.
- Beth and Shayne Dowdie for always believing in me.
- Maggie Landes, MD, for your medical prowess, advice, and critiques—and for your non-diet advocacy in the medical world.
- Erin K. Bowers, PhD, for your insight as a pastor and knowledge as a theologian. I love your passion for keeping diet culture out of the church.
- Reverend Jessica Morris, MDiv, for your spiritual guidance, scriptural knowledge, and continued support.
- Rebecca Greer, MS, RDN, for being such a wonderful human, colleague, and honest early reader of the manuscript.
- Karen Yates for supporting me through one-on-one author coaching.
- My Christian RD group for your constant prayers and encouragement.

Words are inadequate to describe my gratitude for my agent, Rachelle Gardner, of Gardner Literary. I tried to find the right agent for a very long time. Sometimes I ask God to make things easier for me to discern or send me a "God smack." The day after I submitted my query to you, Rachelle, you responded with, "You could not have sent this to a person more likely to read it and love it. I am all the way here for it." Your reply was my God smack. I knew I had found the right fit. Thank you for your wisdom in preparing my proposal and helping me land an equally "here for it" publisher.

I am so thankful to my editor Carolyn McCready, associate publisher Carly Kellerman, and the entire Zondervan / HarperCollins Christian Publishing team for making *Feed Yourself* a reality. I pray that your trust in me and commitment to this message will bring many people food and body freedom, especially in the safe places.

Recommended Reading

The following list of books about diet culture, the church, trauma, and more is not exhaustive. The fruit of twenty years of unlearning and relearning would result in a very long list! This is simply a small sampling of books I've found helpful.

Brooks, Sumner, and Amee Severson. *How to Raise an Intuitive Eater: Raising the Next Generation with Food and Body Confidence*. New York: St. Martin's Essentials, 2022.

Brown, Harriet. *Body of Truth: How Science, History, and Culture Drive Our Obsession with Weight—and What We Can Do about It*. Boston: Da Capo Lifelong, 2015.

Connolly, Jess. *Breaking Free from Body Shame: Dare to Reclaim What God Has Named Good*. Grand Rapids: Zondervan, 2021.

Gordon, Aubrey. *What We Don't Talk about When We Talk about Fat*. Boston: Beacon, 2021.

———. *"You Just Need to Lose Weight": And 19 Other Myths about Fat People*. Boston: Beacon, 2023.

Harrison, Christy. *Anti-Diet: Reclaim Your Time, Money, Well-Being, and Happiness through Intuitive Eating*. New York: Little, Brown Spark, 2021.

King, Chrissy. *The Body Liberation Project: How Understanding Racism and Diet Culture Helps Cultivate Joy and Build Collective Freedom*. New York: Tiny Reparations, 2023.

Kite, Lindsay, and Lexie Kite. *More Than a Body: Your Body Is an Instrument, Not an Ornament*. New York: Houghton Mifflin Harcourt, 2021.

Langberg, Diane. *Redeeming Power: Understanding Authority and Abuse in the Church*. Grand Rapids: Brazos, 2020.

McBride, Hillary L. *The Wisdom of Your Body: Finding Healing, Wholeness, and Connection through Embodied Living*. Grand Rapids: Brazos, 2021.

Perry, Bruce D., and Oprah Winfrey. *What Happened to You? Conversations on Trauma, Resilience, and Healing*. New York: Flatiron, 2021.

Scritchfield, Rebecca. *Body Kindness: Transform Your Health from the Inside Out—and Never Say Diet Again*. New York: Workman, 2016.

Sole-Smith, Virginia. *The Eating Instinct: Food Culture, Body Image, and Guilt in America*. New York: Holt, 2018.

Strings, Sabrina. *Fearing the Black Body: The Racial Origins of Fat Phobia*. New York: New York University Press, 2019.

Tawwab, Nedra Glover. *Set Boundaries, Find Peace: A Guide to Reclaiming Yourself*. New York: TarcherPerigee, 2021.

Taylor, Sonya Renee. *The Body Is Not an Apology: The Power of Radical Self-Love*. 2nd ed. Oakland, CA: Berrett-Koehler, 2021.

Tribole, Evelyn. *Intuitive Eating for Every Day: 365 Daily Practices and Inspirations to Rediscover the Pleasures of Eating*. San Francisco: Chronicle Prism, 2021.

Tribole, Evelyn, and Elyse Resch. *Intuitive Eating: A Revolutionary Program That Works*. 4th ed. New York: St. Martin's Essentials, 2020.

van der Kolk, Bessel. *The Body Keeps the Score: Brain, Mind, and Body in the Healing of Trauma*. New York: Penguin, 2014.

Wolf, Naomi. *The Beauty Myth: How Images of Beauty Are Used against Women*. New York: Harper Perennial, 2002.

Notes

Introduction

1. "Cognitive Dissonance," *Psychology Today*, www.psychologytoday.com/us/basics/cognitive-dissonance#:~:text, accessed November 17, 2022.

Chapter 2: Diet Culture Isn't in the "Safe" Places

1. Christy Harrison, *Anti-Diet: Reclaim Your Time, Money, Well-Being, and Happiness through Intuitive Eating* (New York: Little, Brown Spark 2019), 3.
2. See Sabrina Strings, *Fearing the Black Body: The Racial Origins of Fat Phobia* (New York: New York University Press, 2019).
3. "The $72 Billion Weight Loss and Diet Control Market in the United States, 2019–2023," Business Wire, February 25, 2019, www.businesswire.com/news/home/20190225005455/en/72-Billion-Weight-Loss-Diet-Control-Mar.
4. See Jeffrey M. Hunger, Joslyn P. Smith, and A. Janet Tomiyama, "An Evidence-Based Rationale for Adopting Weight-Inclusive Health Policy," *Social Issues and Policy Review* 14, no. 1 (January 2020): 73–107, https://spssi.onlinelibrary.wiley.com/doi/abs/10.1111/sipr.12062.
5. "Max Lucado—Courage for Today and Hope for Tomorrow," *Dream Big Podcast*, September 29, 2021, www.accessmore

.com/episode/Max-Lucado---Courage-for-Today-and-Hope
-for-Tomorrow.

Chapter 3: It's Simple! Calories In, Calories Out

1. See Ellen A. Wartella, Alice H. Lichtenstein, and Caitlin
   S. Boon, eds., "History of Nutrition Labeling," in *Front-
   of-Package Nutrition Rating Systems and Symbols: Phase
   1 Report* (Washington, DC: National Academies Press,
   2010), www.ncbi.nlm.nih.gov/books/NBK209859, accessed
   November 22, 2022.
2. "Changes to the Nutrition Facts Label," U.S. Food and Drug
   Administration, www.fda.gov/food/food-labeling-nutrition
   /changes-nutrition-facts-label, accessed November 22, 2022.
3. See "Guidance for Industry: Guide for Developing and Using
   Data Bases for Nutrition Labeling," U.S. Food and Drug
   Administration, March 1998, www.fda.gov/regulatory
   -information/search-fda-guidance-documents/guidance
   -industry-guide-developing-and-using-data-bases-nutrition
   -labeling.
4. See Edoardo Capuano et al., "Role of the Food Matrix and
   Digestion on Calculation of the Actual Energy Content of
   Food," *Nutrition Reviews* 76, no. 4 (April 1, 2018): 274–89,
   https://pubmed.ncbi.nlm.nih.gov/29529265.
5. See M. Judith Sánchez-Peña, "Calculating the Metabolizable
   Energy of Macronutrients: A Critical Review of Atwater's
   Results," *Nutrition Reviews* 75, no. 1 (January 2017): 37–48,
   https://pubmed.ncbi.nlm.nih.gov/27974598.
6. See Kevin D. Hall et al., "The Energy Balance Model of
   Obesity: Beyond Calories In, Calories Out," *American
   Journal of Clinical Nutrition* 115, no. 5 (May 2022): 1243–
   54, https://pubmed.ncbi.nlm.nih.gov/35134825.
7. See Leah M. Kalm and Richard D. Semba, "They Starved So
   That Others Be Better Fed: Remembering Ancel Keys and

the Minnesota Experiment," *Journal of Nutrition* 135, no. 6 (June 2005): 1347–52, https://academic.oup.com/jn /article/135/6/1347/4663828.

8. See Kalm and Semba, "They Starved"; Ancel Keys et al., "Experimental Starvation in Man," Air Force Office of Scientific Research, October 15, 1945, https://apps.dtic.mil /sti/citations/ADA473351.

9. See Kalm and Semba, "They Starved."

10. See Kalm and Semba, "They Starved"; Keys et al., "Experimental Starvation in Man."

11. See Courtney C. Simpson and Suzanne E. Mazzeo, "Calorie Counting and Fitness Tracking Technology: Associations with Eating Disorder Symptomatology," *Eating Behaviors* 26 (August 2017): 89–92, https://pubmed.ncbi.nlm.nih.gov /28214452.

12. See Marie Galmiche et al., "Prevalence of Eating Disorders over the 2000–2018 Period: A Systematic Literature Review," *American Journal of Clinical Nutrition* 109, no. 5 (May 2019): 1402–13, https://pubmed.ncbi.nlm.nih.gov/31051507.

Chapter 4: Health Equals Diet and Exercise

1. "Health and Well-Being," World Health Organization, www .who.int/data/gho/data/major-themes/health-and-well-being, accessed November 22, 2022.

2. "Privilege," Wiktionary, https://en.wiktionary.org/wiki /privilege, accessed November 22, 2022.

3. "About Social Determinants of Health," Centers for Disease Control and Prevention, www.cdc.gov/socialdeterminants /about.html, accessed November 22, 2022.

4. "Social Determinants of Health," World Health Organization, www.who.int/health-topics/social-determinants-of-health #tab=tab_1, accessed November 22, 2022.

5. "Social Determinants of Health," U.S. Department of Health

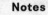

and Human Services, https://health.gov/healthypeople
/objectives-and-data/social-determinants-health, accessed
November 22, 2022.

6. Did you know that people who have experienced food
insecurity are prone to struggling with disordered eating—
particularly binge eating and compensatory behaviors such
as fasting, restriction, meal skipping, laxative/diuretic use,
and purging? Compared to those who are food secure, food-
insecure persons have a greater risk of suffering from binge
eating disorder and bulimia nervosa (see Vivienne M. Hazzard
et al., "Food Insecurity and Eating Disorders: A Review of
Emerging Evidence," *Current Psychiatry Reports* 22, no. 12
[October 30, 2020]: 74, https://pubmed.ncbi.nlm.nih.go
/33125614).

7. See "Social Determinants of Health," World Health
Organization.

8. Cited in "Adverse Childhood Experiences (ACEs)," Centers
for Disease Control and Prevention, www.cdc.gov/vitalsigns
/aces, accessed November 22, 2022.

9. See Vincent J. Felitti et al., "Relationship of Childhood
Abuse and Household Dysfunction to Many of the Leading
Causes of Death in Adults: The Adverse Childhood
Experiences (ACE) Study," *American Journal of Preventive
Medicine* 14, no. 4 (May 1998): 245–58, https://pubmed
.ncbi.nlm.nih.gov/9635069.

10. "Adverse Childhood Experiences (ACEs)."

11. "11 Months before His Assassination, MLK Talks 'New
Phase' of Civil Rights Struggle," NBC News, April 4, 2018,
www.nbcnews.com/video/martin-luther-king-jr-speaks-with
-nbc-news-11-months-before-assassination-1202163779741;
see also www.youtube.com/watch?v=3xD8vWQJEok.

Chapter 5: It's Not a Diet—It's a Lifestyle

1. See Kelly Cuccolo et al., "Intermittent Fasting Implementation and Association with Eating Disorder Symptomatology," *Eating Disorders* 30, no. 5 (2022): 471–91, www.tandfonline.com/doi /full/10.1080/10640266.2021.1922145.

2. See Lauren Reba-Harrelson et al., "Patterns and Prevalence of Disordered Eating and Weight Control Behaviors in Women Ages 25–45," *Eating and Weight Disorders* 14 (2009): e190– e198, https://link.springer.com/article/10.1007/BF03325116; see also "Three Out of Four American Women Have Disordered Eating, Survey Suggests," *ScienceDaily*, April 23, 2008, www.sciencedaily.com/releases/2008/04/080422202514.htm.

3. See Thomas M. Dunn and Steven Bratman, "On Orthorexia Nervosa: A Review of the Literature and Proposed Diagnostic Criteria," *Eating Behaviors* 21 (April 2016): 11–17, www.sciencedirect.com/science/article/abs/pii /S1471015315300362?via%3Dihub; "Orthorexia," NEDA, www.nationaleatingdisorders.org/learn/by-eating-disorder /other/orthorexia, accessed November 22, 2022.

Chapter 6: Your Weight Is the Most Important Indicator of Your Health

1. See A. Janet Tomiyama et al., "How and Why Weight Stigma Drives the Obesity 'Epidemic' and Harms Health," *BMC Medicine* 16, no. 123 (2018), https://bmcmedicine .biomedcentral.com/articles/10.1186/s12916-018-1116-5.

2. See Rebecca M. Puhl and Chelsea A. Heuer, "The Stigma of Obesity: A Review and Update," *Obesity* 17, no. 5 (May 2009): 941–64.

3. Tomiyama, "How and Why Weight Stigma Drives the Obesity 'Epidemic.'"

4. Jeffrey M. Hunger, Joslyn P. Smith, and A. Janet Tomiyama, "An Evidence-Based Rationale for Adopting Weight-Inclusive Health Policy," *Social Issues and Policy Review* 14, no. 1

(January 2020): 73–107, https://spssi.onlinelibrary.wiley.com
/doi/10.1111/sipr.12062.

5. See Traci Mann et al., "Medicare's Search for Effective
   Obesity Treatments: Diets Are Not the Answer," *American
   Psychologist* 62, no. 3 (April 2007): 220–33, https://pubmed
   .ncbi.nlm.nih.gov/17469900.

6. Cited in Mann, "Medicare's Search for Effective Obesity
   Treatments."

7. See A. Janet Tomiyama, Britt Ahlstrom, and Traci Mann,
   "Long-Term Effects of Dieting: Is Weight Loss Related to
   Health?" *Social and Personality Psychology Compass* 7, no. 12
   (December 2013): 861–77, https://compass.onlinelibrary
   .wiley.com/doi/abs/10.1111/spc3.12076.

8. See Tomiyama, "How and Why Weight Stigma Drives the
   Obesity 'Epidemic.'"

9. See Jean-Pierre Montani, Yves Schutz, and Abdul G.
   Dulloo, "Dieting and Weight Cycling as Risk Factors for
   Cardiometabolic Diseases: Who Is Really at Risk?" *Obesity
   Reviews* 16, no. S1 (February 2015): 7–18, https://onlinelibrary
   .wiley.com/doi/10.1111/obr.12251.

10. See Huajie Zou et al., "Association between Weight Cycling
    and Risk of Developing Diabetes in Adults: A Systematic
    Review and Meta-Analysis," *Journal of Diabetes Investigation*
    12, no. 4 (April 2021): 625–32, https://onlinelibrary.wiley
    .com/doi/full/10.1111/jdi.13380.

11. See Jeffrey M. Hunger et al., "Weighed Down by Stigma:
    How Weight-Based Social Identity Threat Contributes
    to Weight Gain and Poor Health," *Social and Personality
    Psychology Compass* 9, no. 6 (June 2015): 255–68, https://
    compass.onlinelibrary.wiley.com/doi/abs/10.1111/spc3.12172.

12. See Kristen M. Lee, Jeffrey M. Hunger, and A. Janet
    Tomiyama, "Weight Stigma and Health Behaviors: Evidence
    from the Eating in America Study," *International Journal of*

Obesity 45 (May 2021): 1499–1509, www.nature.com
/articles/s41366-021-00814-5.

13. See Glenn A. Gaesser and Siddhartha S. Angadi, "Obesity
Treatment: Weight Loss versus Increasing Fitness and
Physical Activity for Reducing Health Risks," *iScience* 24, no.
10 (September 20, 2021): 102995, https://pubmed.ncbi.nlm
.nih.gov/34755078.

14. Cited in Brittany Wong, "PSA: You Probably Don't Need to Be
Weighed at the Doctor's Office," HuffPost, January 19, 2022,
www.huffpost.com/entry/you-dont-need-to-get-weighed-at
-the-doctors-office_l_61e72664e4b05645a6ed73ce.

Chapter 7: Your BMI Is a Problem

1. Aubrey Gordon, *What We Don't Talk about When We Talk
about Fat* (Boston: Beacon, 2020).

2. See Frank Q. Nuttall, "Body Mass Index: Obesity, BMI, and
Health: A Critical Review," *Nutrition Today* 50, no. 3 (May
2015): 117–28, https://pubmed.ncbi.nlm.nih.gov/27340299.

3. Gordon, *What We Don't Talk About*, 49.

4. See Nuttall, "Body Mass Index."

5. Cited in A. Janet Tomiyama et al., "Misclassification of
Cardiometabolic Health When Using Body Mass Index
Categories in NHANES 2005–2012," *International Journal
of Obesity* 40 (February 2016): 883–86, www.nature.com
/articles/ijo201617.

6. See Tomiyama, "Misclassification of Cardiometabolic
Health."

7. Cited in "Eating Disorder Statistics," ANAD, https://anad
.org/eating-disorders-statistics, accessed November 22, 2022.

8. See Cassandra Vanderwall et al., "BMI Is a Poor Predictor of
Adiposity in Young Overweight and Obese Children," *BMC
Pediatrics* 17, no. 1 (June 2, 2017): 135, https://pubmed
.ncbi.nlm.nih.gov/28577356; Charlotte M. Wright et al.,

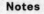

"Body Composition Data Show That High BMI Centiles Overdiagnose Obesity in Children Aged under 6 Years," *American Journal of Clinical Nutrition* 116, no. 1 (July 2022): 122–31, https://academic.oup.com/ajcn/article/116 /1/122/6490122.

9. See Kristine A. Madsen et al., "Effect of School-Based Body Mass Index Reporting in California Public Schools: A Randomized Clinical Trial," *JAMA Pediatrics* 175, no. 3 (March 1, 2021): 251–59, https://pubmed.ncbi.nlm.nih.gov /33196797.

10. Morten Nordmo, Yngvild Sørebø Danielsen, and Magnus Nordmo, "The Challenge of Keeping It Off: A Descriptive Systematic Review of High-Quality, Follow-Up Studies of Obesity Treatments," *Obesity Reviews* 21, no. 1 (January 2020): e12949, https://pubmed.ncbi.nlm.nih.gov/31675146; Tracy L. Tylka et al., "The Weight-Inclusive versus Weight-Normative Approach to Health: Evaluating the Evidence for Prioritizing Well-Being over Weight Loss," *Journal of Obesity* (2014): 983495, https://pubmed.ncbi.nlm.nih.gov/25147734.

11. See Howard Rosen, "Is Obesity a Disease or a Behavior Abnormality? Did the AMA Get It Right?" *Missouri Medicine* 111, no. 2 (March–April 2014): 104–8, https:// pubmed.ncbi.nlm.nih.gov/30323513.

12. See Tylka, "Weight-Inclusive versus Weight-Normative Approach"; Rosen, "Is Obesity a Disease or a Behavior Abnormality?"

13. Shared with me in a personal conversation.

14. "Food Psych #171: Healthcare without Diet Culture with Jennifer Gaudiani," *Food Psych* podcast, October 22, 2018, https://christyharrison.com/foodpsych/6/healthcare -without-diet-culture-with-jennifer-gaudiani.

Chapter 9: Your Weight Secures Your Righteousness

1. See Gerald A. Dienel, "Brain Glucose Metabolism: Integration of Energetics with Function," *Physiological Reviews* 99, no. 1 (January 1, 2019): 949–1045, https://pubmed.ncbi.nlm.nih.gov/30565508.

Chapter 10: We're All Just Gluttons in the Temple

1. Gordon Fee, *The First Epistle to the Corinthians*, New International Commentary on the New Testament (Grand Rapids: Eerdmans, 2014), 292; N. T. Wright, *Paul for Everyone: 1 Corinthians* (Louisville, KY: Westminster John Knox, 2004), 71–72.

2. Shared with me in a personal conversation.

Chapter 11: You Can Feed Yourself

1. See Dorota Myszkowska et al., "Non-IgE Mediated Hypersensitivity to Food Products or Food Intolerance: Problems of Appropriate Diagnostics," *Medicina* 57, no. 11 (November 2021): 1245, www.mdpi.com/1648-9144 /57/11/1245; Catherine Hammond and Jay A. Lieberman, "Unproven Diagnostic Tests for Food Allergy," *Immunology and Allergy Clinics of North America* 38, no. 1 (February 2018): 153–63, https://pubmed.ncbi.nlm.nih.gov/29132671.

Chapter 12: You Can Value Your Physical Health without Dieting

1. See Stephen O'Rahilly and I. Sadaf Farooqi, "Genetics of Obesity," *Philosophical Transactions of the Royal Society of London. Series B Biological Sciences* 361, no. 1471 (July 29, 2006): 1095–1105, https://pubmed.ncbi.nlm.nih.gov /16815794.

2. See Tracy L. Tylka et al., "The Weight-Inclusive versus Weight-Normative Approach to Health: Evaluating the Evidence for Prioritizing Well-Being over Weight Loss,"

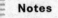

Journal of Obesity (2014): 983495, https://pubmed.ncbi.nlm
.nih.gov/25147734.

3. See Dawn Clifford et al., "Impact of Non-Diet Approaches
on Attitudes, Behaviors, and Health Outcomes: A Systematic
Review," *Journal of Nutritional Education and Behavior* 47,
no. 2 (March–April 2015): 143–55, https://pubmed.ncbi.nlm
.nih.gov/25754299.

4. Katja Rowell, Instagram stories, March 3, 2022, 5:08 p.m.
Used with permission.

5. Suzanne M. Bertisch et al., "Insomnia with Objective Short
Sleep Duration and Risk of Incident Cardiovascular Disease
and All-Cause Mortality: Sleep Heart Health Study," *Sleep*
41, no. 6 (June 1, 2018): zsy047, https://pubmed.ncbi.nlm
.nih.gov/29522193.

6. See Bin Yan et al., "Objective Sleep Efficiency Predicts
Cardiovascular Disease in a Community Population: The
Sleep Heart Health Study," *Journal of the American Heart
Association* 10, no. 7 (April 6, 2021): e016201, https://
pubmed.ncbi.nlm.nih.gov/33719504.

7. See Vaughn W. Barry et al., "Fitness vs. Fatness on All-Cause
Mortality: A Meta-Analysis," *Progress in Cardiovascular
Diseases* 56, no. 4 (January–February 2014): 382–90, https://
pubmed.ncbi.nlm.nih.gov/24438729.

8. See Glenn A. Gaesser and Siddhartha S. Angadi, "Obesity
Treatment: Weight Loss versus Increasing Fitness and
Physical Activity for Reducing Health Risks," *iScience* 24,
no. 10 (September 2021): 102995, https://pubmed.ncbi.nlm
.nih.gov/34755078.

Chapter 14: Mental Health Is Vital to Overall Health and Well-Being

1. Cited in "Mental Illness," National Institute of Mental
Health, www.nimh.nih.gov/health/statistics/mental-illness,
accessed November 22, 2022.

2. Virginia E. Horigian, Renae D. Schmidt, and Daniel J. Feaster, "Loneliness, Mental Health, and Substance Use among U.S. Young Adults during COVID-19," *Journal of Psychoactive Drugs* 53, no. 1 (January–March 2021): 1–9, https://pubmed.ncbi.nlm.nih.gov/33111650.

3. Julianne Holt-Lunstad, Timothy B. Smith, and J. Bradley Layton, "Social Relationships and Mortality Risk: A Meta-Analytic Review," *PLoS Medicine* 7, no. 7 (July 27, 2010): e1000316, https://pubmed.ncbi.nlm.nih.gov/20668659.

4. Cited in Bruno Silva Andrade et al., "Long-COVID and Post-COVID Health Complications: An Up-to-Date Review on Clinical Conditions and Their Possible Molecular Mechanisms," *Viruses* 13, no. 4 (April 18, 2021): 700, https://pubmed.ncbi.nlm.nih.gov/33919537.

5. See Sean F. Woodward et al., "Anxiety, Post-COVID-19 Syndrome-Related Depression, and Suicidal Thoughts in COVID-19 Survivors: Cross-Sectional Study," *JMIR Formative Research* 6, no. 10 (October 25, 2022): e36656, https://pubmed.ncbi.nlm.nih.gov/35763757.

6. See "Depression," National Institute of Mental Health, www.nimh.nih.gov/health/topics/depression#part_2255, accessed November 22, 2022.

7. Patrick Pössel et al., "Do Trust-Based Beliefs Mediate the Associations of Frequency of Private Prayer with Mental Health? A Cross-Sectional Study," *Journal of Religion and Health* 53 (2014): 904–16, https://link.springer.com/article/10.1007/s10943-013-9688-z.

8. See James W. Anderson and Paige A. Nunnelley, "Private Prayer Associations with Depression, Anxiety and Other Health Conditions: An Analytical Review of Clinical Studies," *Postgraduate Medicine* 128, no. 7 (September 2016): 635–41, https://pubmed.ncbi.nlm.nih.gov/27452045.

9. See Sy Atezaz Saeed, Karlene Cunningham, and Richard M. Bloch, "Depression and Anxiety Disorders: Benefits of

Exercise, Yoga, and Meditation," *American Family Physician* 99, no. 10 (May 15, 2019): 620–27, https://pubmed.ncbi.nlm .nih.gov/31083878.

10. See Jeffrey Lambert et al., "Taking a One-Week Break from Social Media Improves Well-Being, Depression, and Anxiety: A Randomized Controlled Trial," *Cyberpsychology, Behavior, and Social Networking* 25, no. 5 (May 10, 2022): 287–93, www.liebertpub.com/doi/10.1089/cyber.2021.0324.

Chapter 17: You Will Not Look like the Influencer, Even If They Say So

1. See Nancy Ellis-Ordway and Virginia Ramseyer Winter, "Weight Stigma as a Violation of the NASW Code of Ethics: A Call to Action," *International Journal of Social Work Values and Ethics* 19, no. 1 (2022), https://jswve.org/volume -19/issue-1/item-09; "Code of Ethics for the Nutrition and Dietetics Profession," Academy of Nutrition and Dietetics, 2018, www.eatrightpro.org/-/media/files/eatrightpro /practice/code-of-ethics/codeofethicshandout.pdf; "AMA Code of Medical Ethics," American Medical Association, revised June 2001, www.ama-assn.org/sites/ama-assn.org /files/corp/media-browser/principles-of-medical-ethics.pdf.

Chapter 18: You Can Detox from Social Media and Trackers

1. Rachel Cohen, Toby Newton-John, and Amy Slater, "The Relationship between *Facebook* and *Instagram* Appearance-Focused Activities and Body Image Concerns in Young Women," *Body Image* 23 (October 2017): 183–87, www.kcl .ac.uk/mental-health-and-psychological-sciences/assets /cohen-et-al-2017.pdf.

2. See Marika Tiggemann and Isabella Barbato, "'You Look Great!': The Effect of Viewing Appearance-Related Instagram Comments on Women's Body Image," *Body Image*

27 (December 2018): 61–66, https://pubmed.ncbi.nlm.nih
.gov/30138768.

3. See Jaime E. Sidani et al., "The Association between Social
   Media Use and Eating Concerns among U.S. Young Adults,"
   Journal of the Academy of Nutrition and Dietetics 116, no. 9
   (September 2016): 1465–72, https://pubmed.ncbi.nlm.nih
   .gov/27161027.

4. Cheri A. Levinson, Laura Fewell, and Leigh C. Brosof, "My
   Fitness Pal Calorie Tracker Usage in the Eating Disorders,"
   Eating Behaviors 27 (December 2017): 14–16, https://
   pubmed.ncbi.nlm.nih.gov/28843591.

5. Jake Linardon and Mariel Messer, "My Fitness Pal Usage
   in Men: Associations with Eating Disorder Symptoms and
   Psychosocial Impairment," *Eating Behaviors* 33 (April 2019):
   13–17, https://pubmed.ncbi.nlm.nih.gov/30772765.

Chapter 19: You Are You on Purpose

1. See "WHO Coronavirus (COVID-19) Dashboard," World
   Health Organization, https://covid19.who.int, accessed
   December 26, 2022.